CREAT

MOVEMENT

& DANCE

IN GROUPWORK

Dedication

This book is dedicated to my mother, Hazel Payne, with blessings, for giving me something of her love for dance.

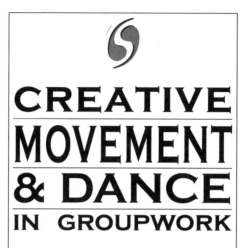

CREATIVE
MOVEMENT
& DANCE
IN GROUPWORK

Helen Payne

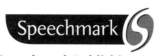

Speechmark Publishing Ltd
Telford Road • Bicester • Oxon OX26 4LQ • UK

Published by
Speechmark Publishing Ltd, Telford Road, Bicester, Oxon OX26 4LQ,
United Kingdom
www.speechmark.net

Illustrations: Bryony & Kirsty Stevens, © Speechmark Publishing 1990

002-0357/Printed in Great Britain/1010

British Library Cataloguing in Publication Data
Payne, Helen
    Creative movement & dance in groupwork. – (Creative activities series)
    1. Dance therapy   2. Social group work
    I. Title
    615.8'5155

ISBN 0 86388 473 3
(Previously published by Winslow Press Ltd under ISBN 0 86388 080 0)

CONTENTS

HELEN PAYNE MPhil has been one of the leading pioneers in dance movement therapy in the United Kingdom. In 1971 she began working in movement and play with adults and children with profound learning difficulties in a hospital setting while attending a specialist physical education course. She went on to work for nine years in special education and with young people labelled 'delinquent'. She has been leading groups for 14 years. Her further professional studies embrace training in dance, special education, counselling and analytical groupwork. She has held lecturing posts on BEd and postgraduate courses specialising in dance and rehabilitation.

Past course leader for the first validated training in DMT at the University of Hertfordshire, she is now a Senior Lecturer in counselling in addition to training dance movement therapists. Her publications include 'The Use of Dance Movement Therapy with Troubled Youth', in Schaefer C (Ed), *Innovative Inventions in Child and Adolescent Therapy* (1988) and numerous papers. Her MPhil (University of Manchester) was the first degree awarded for research in Dance Movement Therapy in the country. Helen is accredited by the Association of Humanistic Practitioners (AHPP), and is a PhD candidate.

FOREWORD

This book is a very special gift for teachers and anyone else who works with personal growth and development. The activities, which reflect the author's sensitive awareness, are practical and easily adapted. More than this, the spirit of the book is what makes it so special; Helen Payne has an obvious love for the Dancing Spirit inside each of us.

I have been a teacher, counsellor and therapist for over thirty years, and I wish I had a pound for every adult who has said to me: "I can't dance, I'm too clumsy."; "I can't sing . . . my teacher told me to move my mouth but not let the sounds come out."; "Don't ask me to draw . . . I can't draw an egg!"; "I hate role play, I can't act, I can't bear having people watch me making a fool of myself." If I had all those pounds, I'd be a very rich woman, and I'd use my money to build a school where people enjoyed their natural *rights* to self-expression through dancing and all of the arts; to try to undo some of the damage that engendered all of those 'I can'ts', and to instil in people that wonderful feeling of "Here I am, I'm dancing!" . . . And then I'd ask Helen Payne to come and work there with me.

The damage to self-esteem is done by teachers (and even parents) in the name of producing 'excellence' — the best choir, the most successful play, the most graceful dancing display at the assembly, the child we can be proud of. But what could be more excellent, more graceful, than the exuberance of children being unselfconscious in the celebration of their own natural rhythms and sounds, their songs, their fantasies, their brilliant colours? And how sad that so many grown-ups are afraid to explore those same inborn gifts, because of the restrictions and criticisms they experienced when they were young.

I believe that *Creative Movement and Dance in Groupwork* will help to redress some of these wrongs . . . I wish for all of its readers the joys of natural dance and movement, and the deep satisfaction of awakening these delights in others.

DONNA BRANDES

Therapist, educator, consultant and trainer

ACKNOWLEDGEMENTS

There are many people I would like to thank for their support and inspiration throughout my life, too many to mention by name here. There are some, however, who emerge as particularly influential in the completion of this particular project. My thanks go, firstly, to my partner, Dr Paul Tosey, for his help in the preparation of the manuscript; then to my daughter Sarah Rebecca, for her patience and creative stimulus; the illustrations are of her at different stages of development.

I would like to thank my colleagues in the Association for Dance Movement Therapy, particularly Lynn Crane and Cataline Garvie, the other co-founders, and colleagues at Hertfordshire College of Art and Design. A big thank you to the students, who continue to be a challenge and constant inspiration for my work. Also to Dr Joanna Harris and Patricia Sanderson, who helped me to understand and develop my work in times of darkness.

Finally, I would like to say a special thank you to all the clients in the various hospitals, clinics, special schools and community homes, without whom this book could not have come to fruition. They continue to initiate me and to teach me on my journey.

This book is based on a booklet written by the author in 1982, entitled *Stepping In*, and published by the Association for Dance Movement Therapy: ISBN 0 951025 60 0 (limited to 100 copies).

PREFACE

Who is the book for?

This book has been written because the application of creative movement and dance in groupwork in education (particularly special education), health, social and community settings is increasing rapidly. Many people are new to the area and want to establish some starting-points before using creative movement and dance; and those who have begun may be seeking to reflect on and develop their practice.

The book is written primarily for people without specialist knowledge of creative movement and dance in groupwork who are looking for such starting-points. If you have a professional or practical interest in the educational and therapeutic use of the arts this book may act as one of many guiding lights on your journey.

The book is also intended to be a helpful reference guide for professional practitioners already familiar with running groups. For those who (like me) sometimes feel helpless when working with particularly difficult, disturbed or disabled groups, this book can provide new energy and empowerment; you can do something!

The aims of the book

This is a practical book to refer to frequently: not a textbook or something to be read once from cover to cover, and certainly not an instruction manual. It gives essential information and guidance, but if your aim is to develop further your skills in this medium you are advised to attend professional training courses and read widely (*see Section 4*); reading the book will definitely not make you a dance movement therapist.

Whilst the book is essentially a source of activities, it also emphasises the need to reflect on the work done. I hope, therefore, that use of the activities will be complemented by reference to the other sections of the book. However, the emphasis is on 'good enough' practice at all times and the guidelines presented aim to encourage you to experiment with activities and to act as a spring-board for your own ideas.

It is also important to say that this is not a 'how-to-do-it' manual; it neither defines a correct procedure for using creative movement and dance, nor provides a blueprint for successful work with your own groups. There is no simple 'right way' to practise that guarantees the achievement of goals. This may be valid when applied to the assembly of objects, for example, although the following quotation casts doubt even on that:

> ... what's really angering about instructions of this sort is that they imply there's only one way to put this rotisserie together — their way. And that presumption wipes out all creativity. Actually there are hundreds of ways to put the rotisserie together and when they make you follow just one way without showing you the overall problem the instructions become hard to follow in such a way as not to make mistakes. You lose feeling for the work. And not only that, it's very unlikely that they've told you the best way. (**Robert Pirsig**, *Zen and the Art of Motorcycle Maintenance*, p160, Corgi, London, 1976.)

In work involving human relations, self-awareness and developmental processes, the elements of creativity and feeling that Pirsig refers to are of even greater significance. Leading groups is a matter of finding ways of working with relationships and problems that are unique to each group, leader and setting. As in many complex situations, much depends on how information like that provided in this book is understood and on how well it is adapted. In each situation there are many opportunities and possible pitfalls.

My hope is that this book will give workers and therapists a continued feel for their work and a new confidence in their own way of doing things. If your response, when reading it or applying it to practice, is 'That's right, that's what I'm doing' or 'That's what I wanted to do', then this hope will have been fulfilled. In conclusion, *Creative Movement and Dance in Groupwork* aims to help you to arrive at sound decisions on how to proceed, decisions about which you feel good and which use your own creativity.

The book's contents

The book is written in four sections:

Section 1 gives a brief description of the history and background of movement and dance work. This is the section to read if you want to know how creative movement and dance has come to be used in treatment and rehabilitation, and why and how it is of value.

Section 2 outlines the principles of movement, including developmental movement and Rudolf Laban's movement categorisation. This provides a brief outline of the main theoretical models and tools of creative movement and dance. The section also gives practical advice on the planning, development and evaluation of programmes of dance and movement.

Section 3, which constitutes both the bulk and the heart of the book, describes activities that have been found to be workable with children, adolescents and adults in a variety of settings. A core principle of the book is that action and evaluation proceed simultaneously, so that most activities incorporate suggestions for future development. The activities are open to discussion and modification, to be experimented with and improved upon by you. Some activities can be reviewed in discussion time within the group, further promoting levels of insight and understanding for individuals.

Section 4 gives further information, such as references, a glossary of terms, training courses and other helpful addresses.

Finally, no programme of creative movement and dance can exist in isolation; it needs to relate to the specific problems and strengths of the population you are working with and to the approach of the setting. Nor can a programme exist outside you; what you contribute both personally and professionally will shape the programme's nature and success.

SECTION 1

HISTORICAL BACKGROUND

HISTORICAL BACKGROUND

Introduction

Dance has been part of human life throughout the ages, performed to celebrate, for example, births, marriages, harvests and wars (**Sachs**, 1937). People dance as naturally as they play, court, feed or fight and dance is often used to express those functions. Throughout the world dance is part of our rituals (*see Glossary*) and our heritage. The *Gulbenkian Dance Report* (1980) defined dance as 'part of the history of human movement, part of the history of human culture, and part of the history of human communication'.

Growth, health and creativity are often seen to be interrelated, the potential for all being present in human beings. Improvisation and re-enactment, through dance, of earlier experience, can help to release tension and aid self-expression and integration. In our society, where there is perhaps a declining emphasis on physical work or action, energy is often repressed; hence the popular need for physical outlets such as the leisure pursuits of aerobics and jogging.

Recent research (for example, **Doyne** *et al.*, 1987) has demonstrated that this action of physical doing helps to release tension and depression. Dance and movement are active, body-based, expressive and communicative media, and through them the build-up of adrenalin can be dispersed and aggression, rigidity and apathy can be discharged in a socially acceptable manner. To dance out anger or joy, love or sadness enhances the individual's ability to express these affects. Inaction and depression are often synonymous; the creative act of moving alone or with others can enable an integration of mind, body and spirit.

Leste and Rust (1984) studied the effects of modern dance on anxiety with subjects in further education. Their results indicated a statistically significant drop in scores for anxiety levels in the experimental group in comparison to the music therapy and physical education control groups. A study by **Puretz** (1978) compared the effects of dance and physical education on the self-concept of disadvantaged girls. There was a significant increase in the dance subjects' self-concept. In another study, **May** *et al.* (1978), schizophrenics were shown to benefit from group dance movement therapy.

Other areas of considerable research have been in the fields of body image, movement in space and proximetrics (the body in space and in relationships); for example, studies have been made of the proximity-seeking behaviour of infants and children towards their mother after a period of separation (**Heinicke and Westheimer**, 1966).

3

Historical development

The systematic use of dance and movement in treatment of various kinds, both in the UK and the USA, dates back about half a century. To some extent development in the UK has been separate from that in the United States, although these two strands have always been linked and have become more closely connected over time.

The UK has long had a tradition of including dance as a core educational discipline, especially at primary level. Recognition of the potential for rehabilitation and therapy through dance and movement experiences began in this country in the 1940s, although very little was written about the work at that time.

A significant figure in the development of dance and movement in the UK was Rudolf Laban (1879–1958). His contribution was the systematic categorisation of movement. In dance movement therapy this enables the therapist to use movement observations as both a diagnostic and an assessment element in the work. Laban's analysis and categorisation of movement has added to the other bodies of literature on non-verbal communication. His early thinking on movement therapy is described in an article (1983) written in 1949 when he was working with patients in Exeter. One of Laban's students, Warren Lamb, added to the analysis with a category focussing on shape (**Lamb**, 1979) which evolved out of his work in management training.

Following Laban's analysis of movement and contribution to dance in education, his students and others began to promote the use of dance and movement in treatment and therapeutic contexts. For example, **Sherborne** (1974) and **Wethered and Gardner** (1986) used Laban's contribution as far back as the 1940s. Theorists such as **North** (1972) later added to his ideas, correlating movement with personality traits. Others such as **Bainbridge et al.** (1953) used dance in psychiatry and **Oliver** (1968; 1975) had success using it in hospitals and schools for the mentally handicapped.

In the 1950s education authorities such as the then West Riding and Manchester pioneered the use of Laban's work in their education of teachers and in their primary and secondary schools. They trained primary and specialist secondary teachers of physical education in the application of his ideas to movement and dance education, which stressed creativity and groupwork approaches.

Soon all education authorities were using Laban's principles in their dance and movement education programmes. The child-centred educational philosophy in England at that time helped in the fostering of the work which was endorsed by the Department of Education and Science (**Foster**, 1977) and called 'modern educational dance'.

4

Although Laban was a gifted teacher and had a profound effect on the history and development of creative dance in the UK, the status of his theories has been criticised by, for example, **Gordon Curl** as early as 1967, and by others later. One major source of contention is that some of Laban's writings speak of movement in formal geometrical and arbitrary cosmological terms and do not acknowledge that movement takes place in phenomenal space, within a context. Thus there is scepticism about ascribing expressive meanings to movement, which is not contextualised or qualitatively based, by reference to a preconceived cosmological theory.

America saw the earlier development of a specific therapy using dance and movement, together with the formation of a professional association, the American Dance Therapy Association (ADTA), in 1966. The American literature of the 1960s and 1970s relates the pioneering dance movement therapists' perceptions of the therapeutic process (**Chace**, 1975). Dance and movement experiences were found to help groups of mentally ill and handicapped people in a variety of ways.

In the UK since the 1960s, in isolated pockets, physical educators, special educators, dance educators and artists, social workers, nurses, psychologists, physiotherapists, occupational therapists and others have explored these media with populations (*see Glossary*) such as psychiatric patients, the learning disabled, autistics, young offenders, the elderly, drug users and children 'at risk'.

Dance movement therapists in Britain are now defining professional boundaries and a clear basis for the work is becoming established. However the profession has developed later than the other arts therapies in the UK and dance/movement therapy in America. This has been the result of, for example, practitioners working in isolation, and a lack of written and published evidence of practice.

The Association for Dance Movement Therapy (ADMT) was formally established in 1982 (**Payne**, 1983); among its aims are the promotion of training and education in dance movement therapy (DMT) and the provision of a shared focal point for practitioners in the field.

Dance as movement and dance as performance art

Everyone has a general idea of dance as an art form. For those people relatively new to the field it may be useful to set out the differences between the use of dance as an art form and the use of dance as movement in therapy. DMT grew out of the use of dance and movement with special needs groups but has since become more distinct. It is important to make some of these distinctions clear for those people intending to use this book.

Something that may be puzzling for those new to the arts therapies, but which is an issue of considerable significance for the professions, is the distinction between people working as teachers or artists with special needs groups and those working as therapists. In the field of dance and movement, the former are exemplified by Wolfgang Stange and his calisthenics with the mentally handicapped, and **Levete** (1985), and the latter by those such as **Payne** (1979; 1984) and **Meekums** (1987). Each field has provided new ideas and research.

Movement is the medium for both fields, with its raw materials of the body, time, space and energy or force. When using dance as art it may focus on, for example, performance, exercise or educational aims. However it is the context and underlying assumptions which determine such aims.

Dance as movement is the conceptual approach used in DMT; it ignores aesthetic concerns and its nature is explained in psychological, sociological and historical terms. This approach is a development of the original 'movement' approach to dance common in the 1960s, which then formed the basis for the 'human movement studies' model of the mid-1970s. Then, dance was seen as one example of a movement form amongst many. This is the context for adopting the term 'dance movement therapy' in the UK, in contrast to the term 'dance therapy' or dance/movement therapy which is used in the USA.

The 1980s have seen dance as a performance art extending into educational and community contexts. It is also used with special needs groups. Dance as performance art offers technique and choreography and these relate to modern dance in the theatre. When using dance as a performance art, however, a particular style of movement technique is employed. The form and the technique are derived from a specific body-based training in a style such as ballet, Cunningham, Hawkins, Limon or Graham (**Cohen**, 1966).

Laban's approach, used by therapists and others, emphasises creative dance in which movement is self-generated and linked together, so forming the dance. The components are employed by the mover or therapist for expression or intervention. In this area of creative dance the main points of interest might be, for example, movement qualities, or the relationships between people through body activity in the dance.

The orientation towards either dance as movement or dance as art influences the aims and nature of the session, methods for development, and evaluation procedures; this will be true whether the session is for therapy, education, performance, or some other aim. During creative dance, any form and style present are those the individual chooses to use. Improvisation can lead to a depth in feeling commensurate with the movement process. The mover could begin to work with, for example, reclaiming or reconnecting with specific parts of their body: by becoming more self-aware they may acknowledge imperfections or exert a more positive control over their bodies.

The major difference between dance as a performance art and dance as movement in therapy lies in the basic theory. The central principle of dance movement therapy is that a significant and powerful connection exists between motion and emotion. The role of the therapist is to give attention to the mover, helping them to explore this connection in their own life and experience, with the aim of healing themselves and enriching the relationship between the physical and the psycho-emotional. This movement process is a dance, but as such it does not aim to make 'art' or to use dance for performance. The approach to and context of that dance are significantly different.

This central principle is grounded in knowledge about child development. Long before an infant understands verbal communications or responds to visual cues if feels the subtleties of the mother's physical attentions and of its own movement. These early memories are pre-verbal, since the nervous system is insufficiently developed for the storage of verbal information. The early mother—infant relationship is a symbiotic phase, one of memories pre-verbally stored in the body. Through kinaesthetic sensations, particularly in holding and handling by the mother, the body image, a sense of self and the mind's structure emerge.

There are stage-specific actions which occur throughout the normal development of a child; these include grasping, rolling, rocking, creeping, throwing, crawling, standing, falling, balancing, walking, running, skipping and jumping. Attitudes of family members towards these actions may need to be identified and worked with to free the person from inhibitions experienced in childhood because of, say, negative parental attitudes towards climbing.

Any movement not experienced at the appropriate stage of development because of attitudes or restrictions may be experienced at a later stage, even in an adult body. Over-keen parenting can also damage normal development, as with, for example, pushing a child to walk before crawling has been consolidated. These 'lost' experiences of motoric development can be physicalised through specific structures: for example, sitting to turning to crawling to sitting sequences. The adult may eventually recapture some of the perceptual and emotional processes accompanying such a stage. Therefore a knowledge of the fundamental physical stages in infant—child development can be useful to those of us working, with for example, developmentally delayed groups or those who have become impoverished at a particular stage, for whatever reason.

Thus there are some basic differences between dance performance, creative dance and dance movement therapy; while dance performance and creative dance, like sport, may have therapeutic effects, it does not constitute a therapy because it does not pursue systematically the integration of conscious and unconscious experience. DMT has a clear basis for its therapeutic value. Workers trained in dance as performance with a specific technique can develop into dance movement therapists; indeed some early therapists were typically so trained, more so in America than in the United Kingdom. What is important is that, in DMT, dance skills/technique, dance/movement education and/or performance cease to be the main aim of the work.

A more detailed description of the process of dance movement therapy now follows.

Dance movement therapy: The mode of working

In the course of dance movement therapy, unconsciously derived movement responses can elicit the associational recall and re-enactment of early phenomena, making conscious the imprint of feelings which may be re-experienced and acknowledged at a different level of consciousness.

People can engage deeply in this process by functioning at a non-verbal level, with movement as the medium. Creative dance improvisations and unconscious free associational movement are fundamental to this form of therapy, whether it takes place individually or in groups. By employing expressive approaches such as in Laban's methods and facilitating play in movement and sensory processes, re-experiencing and symbolic enactment enable the pre-verbal experience, however deeply buried, to become explicit.

The client, not the leader, is the one who can create change, although the leader needs to believe in the client's ability to do so. Clients may be encouraged to work in one of two ways during

8

sessions; both ways are spontaneous, self-initiated and self-directed. The first is an 'outside-in', the second an 'inside-out' approach. Improvisation requires a spontaneity of activity, something many groups find difficult. Movement can stir the feelings just as feelings can stir and be reflected in movement. A cautious approach, with carefully selected activities, will be demanded before some groups are confident enough to improvise.

In the first approach the group leader sets a theme, a movement game or a structure, and the group works within that. Movement is often with eyes open and the movement relates to an actual person or object; it aids awareness of emotional patterns which group members establish with others in their immediate environment.

The second approach involves the group in self-initiated movements which arise out of interactions, feelings, and opportunities created in the session for individual work, such as identifying a physical symptom and moving 'as if . . .' This is often done with eyes closed, (opening them at intervals to keep an orientation in the room) and the movement relates only to the internal process as it is being experienced, often as a pre-conscious state. With this second approach, the individuals in the group move to images which emerge spontaneously from within themselves, rather than to any suggestions from the group leader. These images are generated either from bodily-based feelings, from sensations or from the spontaneous movements themselves; the images emerge into awareness and by so doing can help to identify the experience of the mover. This method is more appropriate for 'neurotic' than the more 'psychotic' client groups, since it requires the capacity to bear the tension of opposites (to open fully to the unconscious while maintaining a strong conscious standpoint).

These pre-verbal experiences may then be shared at a verbal level if appropriate, transforming body-felt experiences into thoughts and words (externalising them to others). The changing self may be reflected in the body image which needs to be moved rather than talked through in order to give the individual feedback at the pre-verbal level from their own body and movement. However verbalisation at the right time can be a supportive aspect of the process, as long as it is not overused. The reality orientation of the body work needs to be returned to after such dialogue. Feedback from others helps to encourage new body-felt relationships. Alternatively, different media can be used; for example, sometimes by using drawing or sound-making the movement process can be clarified. To begin to expose the self in moving action can be difficult for some groups; or some individuals in the group; simply being in the space with the group, or the expressing of the 'non-movement' issue through verbal acknowledgement may be major achievements. With other groups the continued need to move all the time may be a defence or resistance to being still, talking or reflecting.

Taking responsibility for one's movement action involves taking responsibility for the self in action and the feelings one has in the process. This can result in a will to change. After acknowledging (owning) the feeling and expressing it in the dance, some communication can then develop within the inner world of the client and finally in the outer world, from self to other.

The area of dance movement as therapy is still embryonic, yet it has been found to be meaningful for a variety of client groups.

Conclusion

This section has given a brief introduction to the part creative dance and movement experiences play in treatment and rehabilitation. Wounds can never heal completely. A person always reflects the fact of having been healed or healing; and dance and movement are not a panacea, certain to produce growth, health or cure. However the group who have danced together will have been assisted towards, for example, becoming more cohesive, more responsive, more aware of their choices, and more courageous.

The aim of dance and movement work is not simply to evoke or reflect feelings, but to encourage the client to begin to feel in expressive action. Working towards acknowledging the body more and reawakening the initial life force enables people to become participants in their own change process.

Finally, as practitioners and group leaders, our own life experience, attitude, beliefs and body state are crucial to our interventions. Our orientation and experiences in dance and movement will affect the programme we create with our groups, as will our relationships with ourselves, with the group and movement processes. Our own dance is the well-spring of inspiration and, as such, needs cherishing.

PRACTICAL & THEORETICAL ISSUES

Developmental movement processes

An understanding of developmental movement can help to give the leader a starting-point for some activities, especially with those groups that have a developmental lag. A developmental movement structure (*see p 8*) may be given in one session or divided and presented sequentially over several sessions. The whole structure may be used on specific stages only. The following is a brief overview of the motoric development which normally takes place in early childhood. Structures which may be used to illuminate and re-create these stages are then built around the process.

Motor patterns

Some people may have criticisms of the stages presented, based upon their own experience; however the patterns shown are those which can generally be expected in normal development. A developing infant may omit some stages altogether, whilst others may need to be consolidated longer. In normal development one thing is certain: physical growth will always take place with accompanying motor patterns. None the less environment and physical opportunity can affect these patterns.

A knowledge of these patterns can enable a worker to provide for consolidation and/or the next stage in motor development, for example with clients who have a developmental lag, or to encourage clients' re-experiencing of specific stages. By referring to the figures you can follow the summary of the motoric stages of development at monthly frequencies.

By one month

At birth the infant can turn its head, focus on objects and usually has flexed limbs, with hands near to the face. It has a strong sucking action, roots for the nipple and shows a grasp in its hands by which it can be lifted. The startle reflex, where both arms shoot outwards if it is shocked or roughly handled, is prevalent, later to be lost, as is the rigid body position when held horizontally.

Drawing 1 shows the infant on its front; it can raise its head slightly.

Drawing 2 shows the infant being held sitting; its head falls backwards.

Drawing 3 shows the infant flexing and extending arms and legs and turning its head from side to side while on its back.

Drawing 4 shows the walking reflex action which is lost soon after birth. The infant will flex and extend its knees alternately when held upright with the sole of the foot on a surface.

Drawing 5 shows the infant raising its pelvis and flexing its knees to make a crawling action, although there is no forward movement as yet.

Drawing 6 shows the infant rolling from its side onto its back, often with the heavy head leading and the back arching.

By two months

Drawing 1 shows the infant on its front, raising its head to 45 degrees and its torso onto its forearms.

Drawing 2 shows the infant being held in a sitting position, where its head wobbles and its back is weak.

By three months

Drawing 1 shows the infant finding and exploring its hands; it is also noticing and touching other body parts, such as its feet. It can involuntarily grasp objects on contact and raises its head forward when held sitting.

Drawing 2 shows the infant's hips extended while it is lying on its back.

By four months

Drawing 1 shows that the infant can now raise its upper torso onto its elbows and lift its head to 90 degrees.

Drawing 2 shows the infant rolling from its back onto its side; it can now hold its back upright when sitting, but it is still weak. It can hold its head up unaided.

By five months

Drawing 1 shows the infant with its hands flat open on the floor as it raises its upper torso, pushing strongly away from the floor. At this stage its grasp is voluntary and it actively aims to reach objects.

Drawing 2 shows the infant supporting itself on its thorax. At this stage it can actively help in postures such as sitting, and extends and flexes all its limbs while exploring body parts (touching its feet, for example).

By one month

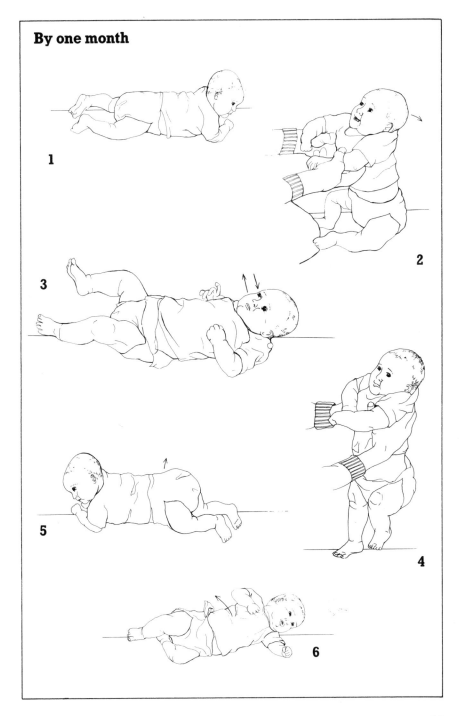

1

2

3

4

5

6

By six months

Drawing 1 shows the infant raised up on its open hands when in the prone position. The head is back and the neck strongly supports it.

Drawing 2 shows the infant lifting its head up and forward when lying on its back, abdominal muscles becoming stronger. At this stage the infant can stand with help (often on tips of toes).

Drawing 3 shows the infant picking up objects with one hand while supporting itself with the other, when prone.

Drawing 4 shows the infant rolling from front to back.

By seven months

Drawing 1 The infant sits upright without support; hands are often forward on the floor to prevent falling.

Drawing 2 shows the infant rolling from its back to its front. Often rocking movements initiate this stage.

Drawing 3 shows the 'letting go' of objects.

By eight months

Drawing 1 shows that the infant can sit alone and has good muscle tones.

Drawing 2 shows the infant rolling in both directions.

Drawing 3 shows the infant rolling itself from lying to sitting.

Drawing 4 shows the infant raising itself from prone to bearing weight on hands and toes. By this stage it may have pushed itself along on its back with its feet, moved around in a circle on its front/back and made swimming/pushing actions while prone.

By nine months

Drawing 1 shows the infant rocking back and forth to begin crawling, often backwards at first.

Drawing 2 shows that the infant needs to hold on to furniture/people to balance in the upright position (hips out behind). Falling occurs frequently at this stage.

By eleven months

Drawing 1 shows that the child can walk while supporting itself on a wide base.

Drawing 2 shows that the child can 'bear walk' on alternate limbs, 'all fours'.

Drawing 3 shows the child holding, then throwing, the ball to an adult. The child can now point at objects.

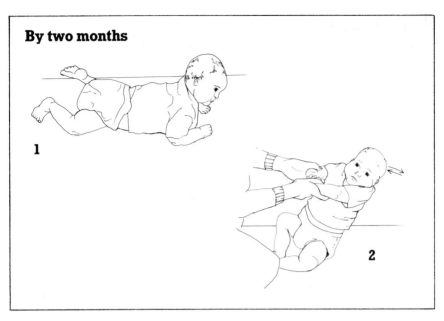

By two months

1

2

By three months

1

2

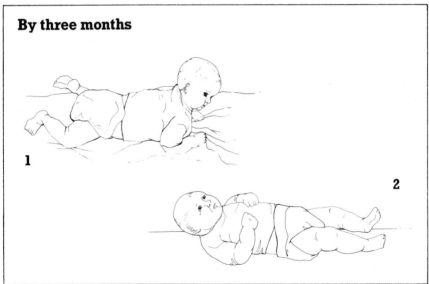

By twelve months

Drawing 1 shows that the child can walk when held with one hand by an adult. The child sits, rolls, crawls, shuffles, stands and falls.

Drawing 2 shows the child bending to pick up a released object.

By four months

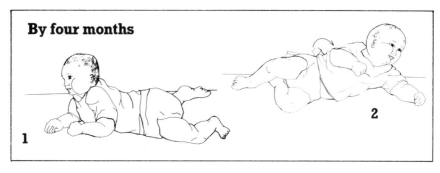

1

2

By five months

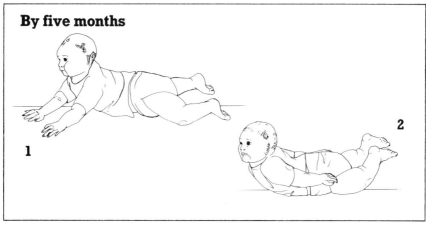

1

2

By six months

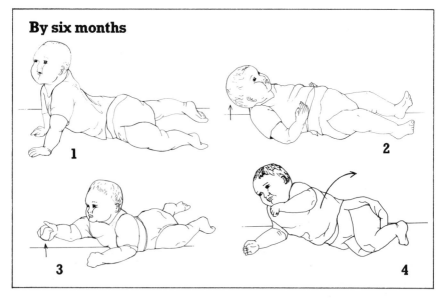

1

2

3

4

By seven months

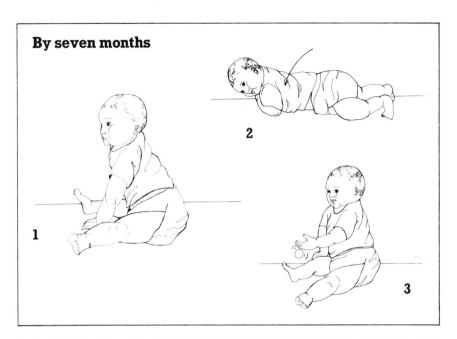

By eight months

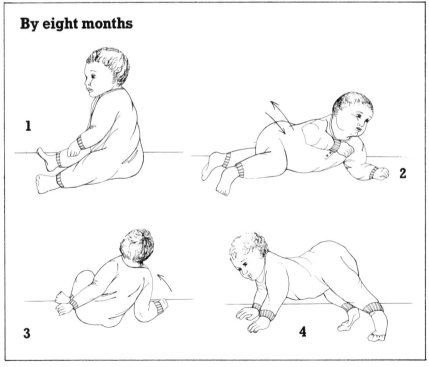

By nine months

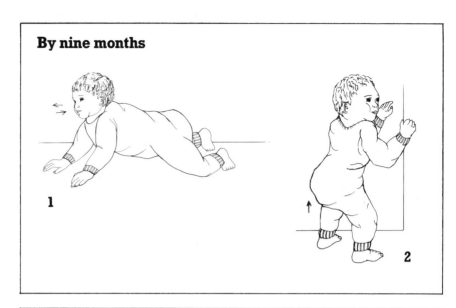

1

2

By eleven months

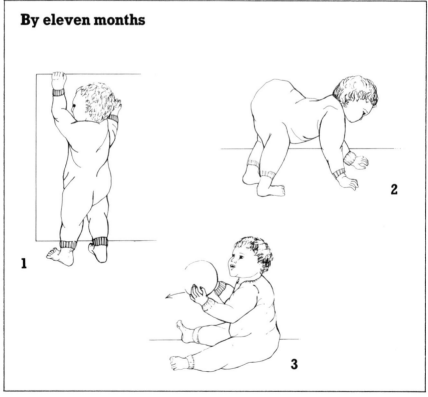

1

2

3

By twelve months

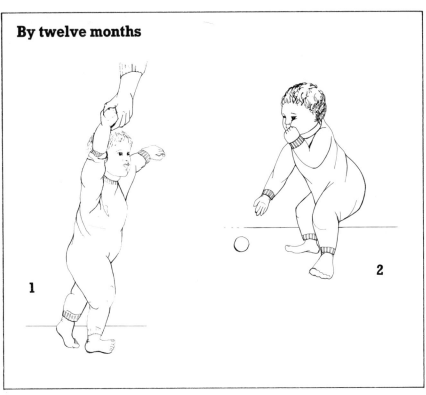

1

2

By fifteen months

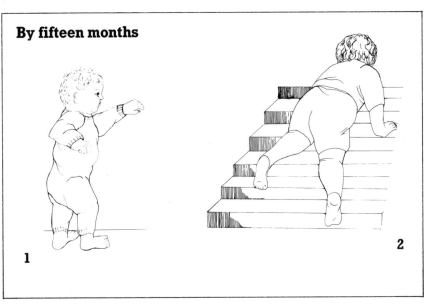

1

2

By eighteen months

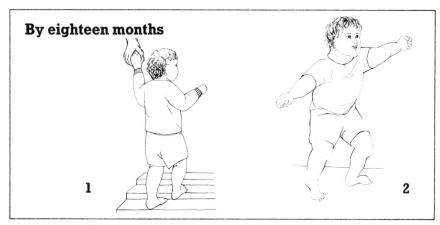

1   2

By two years

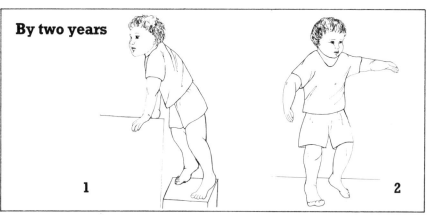

1   2

By three years

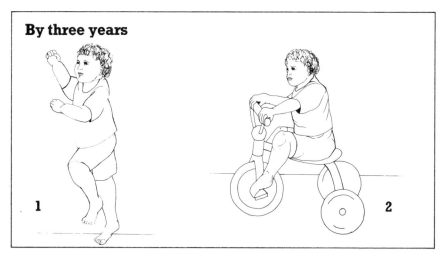

1   2

By fifteen months

Drawing 1 shows the child walking alone on a wide base, arms outstretched.

Drawing 2 shows the child climbing stairs on all fours. The child kneels, stands up, falls. Its balance is poor, although release of objects is more precise; pushing objects begins, as does fine motor development.

By eighteen months

Drawing 1 shows the child climbing stairs with an adult.

Drawing 2 The child runs with a wide base and falls. It can jump with feet together, pull a toy behind, walk backwards, and push a ball with its feet.

By two years

Drawing 1 shows the child climbing.

Drawing 2 shows the child 'dancing'. The child can now balance and jump on both feet, kick a ball, go up and down stairs, run fast, and skip.

By three years

Drawing 1 shows the child jumping on one foot (hop). Balance is now good; it leaps, hops; alternate arms swing in walk.

Drawing 2 shows the young child riding a tricycle.

Possible developmental movement structure A

Use language which will be appropriate for your client group. Please note that this is not designed as a rebirthing experience (*see Glossary*); an in-depth training is required for this — see *section 4*. Feel free to use your own words once you have a sense of the structure.

The leader says:

1 "Become aware of the space in the room, then find a place on the floor you feel comfortable in. Find a way to get down to the floor, then close your eyes."

2 "Find a comfortable curled position. Imagine you are in a perfect environment. You have no needs, and all flows in your movement; your exploration of hands, toes, body is accidental. You turn over, stretch and bend. You are in the womb, getting ready to be born."

3   "This is birth – the first pain in life. You are moving forward and being moved towards a new environment. Your eyes open wide to find that it is bright and noisy, the air is cold, and you cry and breathe alone for the first time. You hear your own sound and your mother's sound in a different way. You rest, very tired."
(Do not spend long in this phase; the purpose of this structure is to experience a range of movements as if for the first time, not to re-live the birth itself.)

4   "Your hands, closed or open, often go to your mouth. You start to make other very small movements, unable to do much. Different body parts move – your back, elbows, knees, hands and feet. You move onto your stomach and feel your contact with the floor. You move your arms and chest, and find that you can push up and away from the floor. You can rock from side to side and forward and back. These are your first attempts at locomotion [*see Glossary*]. Your eyes may be open or closed; whenever they open you look up and out. You can now support your weight with your hands. You kick strongly."

5   "Now you can hold your head up, with the neck muscles much stronger. You experience being upright in this sense. Roll from side to side; this is your first large movement. Now you can start to crawl to get around, and you move to grasp things that attract you. You can change your own environment by locomotion. Can you remember the kind of house you were in when you first crawled? Who was there? You can change from crawling to sitting upright to kneeling to shifting forward on your seat. You use forward, sideways and backwards directions."

6   "Now you can stand while holding onto something, your feet wide apart and very unsteady. Being vertical is a new dimension. Someone helps you walk forward. You test out your mobility and stumble or fall, but are excited at the freedom of movement as you move alone for the first time."

7   "You can now succeed and fail at those first steps. Step, step quickly and grab hold, totter, fall. You choose where to go, explore the environment. Step onto, pull onto, pull through and reach over objects. You practise your walk."

8   "Now as you get older and more confident your walk becomes a run, then, later, a jump with both feet; then continue leaping, hopping, doing somersaults and balances, climbing and skipping. Where are you; at school, with brothers or sisters?"

9   "Notice others but play alongside rather than with them. Perhaps follow or copy a movement. Touch and interact. Test your new-found movements against other peoples.' Try not to talk. Groups form spontaneously — join and leave them, choosing to remain or ignore them and be alone. Where are you at this stage? Can you remember a particular place?"

10 "Now you are 11 to 12 years old, independent yet dependent. You like cuddles still. Your body is beginning to change and you are aware of how you appear to others. How are you moving?"

11 "You are 14 to 16 years old now, frustrated, angry and bored. Who are you? There are big questions in life. Friends and looking alike are very important to you. Your sexual identity is developing. You are neither an adult nor a child. How do you move? What kind of walk do you have? What kind of rhythm does it have?"

12 "You are 16 to 18 years old now, struggling with decisions about boy/girl friends, perhaps your first car and job. You form close friendships; you may feel conflict and rebellion."

13 "At 20 to 30 years you feel safer as you grow and mature. Find your own movement signature — how do you move now? With what preferences? Slowly, quickly, strongly, softly? Lots of factors in your life make up your movement style. Is it work, people, sports, nurturing roles? Allow movement to happen; this could have a repetitive pattern which is like a metaphor for your life. What sound or word or image accompanies it? What colour is it?"

14 "As you get older your rhythm changes; how does the movement change? What are the limitations? Any sound, images? Bones are more fragile, it's not so easy to get up, sit down or find a resting place. You feel satisfied, relaxed. Breathing is easy. Reflect on your life."

15 Group feedback.

Possible developmental movement structure B

1   "Lie on your back in a space as though you were a young infant."

2   "Open out while lying on your back, and make opening and closing movements with your limbs."

3   "Explore your toes and fingers; grasp and release."

4   "Roll over onto your front, allowing the head to lead. Lift the head, push up your chest and rock forward and back."

5 "Pull yourself along, pushing with knees and feet. Push yourself along on your back, using both your feet."

6 "Crawl, creep, sit up, turn and lie down. Repeat this sequence of movements so that they flow one after the other."

7 "Bottom shuffle along, fall forward, backward and sideways, catching yourself with your hands. Change direction of locomotion."

8 "Do 'bear walks' (on all fours, feet and hands in contact with the ground, arms and legs extended)."

9 "Stand up, holding onto a stable object; fall down, fight gravity again, raise your hips and let your weight fall onto your legs."

10 "Climb onto objects, then stand alone as if for the first time."

11 "Take a few first steps alone."

12 "Walk, run, walk, climb and run."

13 "Leap, first from one foot then from both."

14 "Jump with feet together, hop, balance and skip."

15 "Repeat the above but with a partner assisting the movement experiences, for example helping rolls, standing and catching. The partner makes contact with your head (eg. by resting a hand upon it lightly) to ensure that it leads the movement. The partner helps in forward, backward and stretched and curled sideways rolls. For example, support their forward roll by having them roll over your shoulder while you are sitting with legs astride. Help them to curl over and around their centre while you maintain contact with hands on their head and body."

Non-verbal communication as expression and communication within the group

Movement, as a medium for dance, is the expressive and communicative aspect of human development. **Espenak** (1981) elaborates:

> By the term dance we can refer to an entire constellation of physical expression. In so far as movement, gesture or posture, represents communication to the self, leader or group — that movement is dance.

Movement is at the core of our development and has a profound influence on the learning of speech, socially acceptable behaviour and cognitive skills. In this sense we are looking, not at functional movement, that is movement in which a skill is performed as in specific dance techniques, sports or lifting a cup to drink, but at the expressive movement form. Extensive research has been carried out on the observation of movement and its emotional communication; see, for example, **Birdwhistell** (1970), **Condon** (1969), **Lamb** (1979), **North** (1972) and **Hall** (1973). It is this observable relationship between emotion and motion which is expressive of the individual. Body posture, facial grimaces, the strength of a handshake and other movements found in social communication have much in common with creative dance.

Amongst the basic assumptions of using creative dance and movement processes as vehicles for change is that, by changing the body so that it functions differently in movement terms, we promote a corresponding effect on the mind when both are focused on together. **Trudi Schoop** (1973), a well-known early pioneer in dance therapy from California, wrote:

> If I am correct in assuming mind and body are interactive I feel a problem of disturbance can be influenced from either side. When psychoanalysis brings about a change in the mental attitude there should be a corresponding change in body behaviour. And when dance therapy brings about a change in the body there should be a corresponding change in the mind. The approach to verbal therapy is through the mind—body and the approach to dance therapy is through the body—mind. Both methods want to change the whole being. (p 45)

However, we must be cautious about taking for granted a simple mind/body equation, that is assuming that what happens physically happens in an equivalent way in the structure of the human psyche. A person is their body, not the possessor of their body. To change the mind—body is to change the shape of the self. People need to deal adequately with the changing shapes of their lives, a process of continual reorganisation, which **Piaget** (1952) called 'accommodation'. Habitual patterns of movement, frequently based on early pre-verbal experiences, are often the only resource we have to make sense of the world. When we become stuck in those patterns, as in reactive behaviour, learning new behaviours is imperative if we are to grow and integrate changes. When initiating creative action in movement another resource for dealing with life changes is made available. Some patterns we have are no longer relevant to our healthy functioning and need to adapt to our present needs.

The advantage of focusing on the movement behaviour is that the body is often more pliable, plastic and capable of reorganisation than is our thinking. The body does not lie about itself, but we can lie about the body. The body is capable of regenerating, reshaping itself and growing. Changes on a biochemical and neuromuscular level can be initiated by the person themselves; this is the basis of biofeedback techniques.

To alter a life situation is to change not just through the mind alone but through the way the self is used. A change in the body's behaviour can often be facilitated by non-verbal means at a primary level of functioning, that is, at the felt level (**Gendlin**, 1962), allowing an expression of repressed and important emotions. The movement phases alone, as in going through the motions, are not enough in themselves: the emotional aspects must be worked with in conjunction with the physical. Clients who resist movement need to be helped gradually to initiate their own involvement. 'Not moving' or 'stillness' is equally important; it is not necessary to be engaged in gross bodily movement to participate. By observing the subtle, shadowy movements an involvement may result. However small the steps, the leader needs to be sensitive in regard to the way this involvement is developed. The leader's movement range is the resource which enables the participant to move in less accessible directions, levels, dimensions and combinations of qualities, creating and exploring other forms of expression.

Developing creative dance as expression and communication within the group

The raw materials for dance are rhythm and pattern. As discussed above, one could say that any movement is dance — look at slowed down or speeded up film or videotape; a pattern of rhythmical spatial structures can be seen. **Stern** (1979) refers to the choreography between the mother and child.

Movement can be classified into three types: functional or instrumental (as in, for example, picking up a cup to drink, akin to **Allport**'s (1961) coping behaviour); quantitative (as in, for example, running fast in sport); and qualitative (as in the expression of moods and feelings and in expressive and aesthetic qualities). **Sandle** (1975) has discussed these at some length. It is the last type with which we are concerned here, that of the qualitative dynamics of movement.

To find a movement is success enough for some clients; making it into a dance may be too difficult because of their level of functioning. Thus we need to work developmentally, going from simple movement play and developmental processes (*see pp 13 – 26*) towards symbolic movement and communicative dance. When developing the group's movement it may be possible for them to improvise, then select and link movements together. Once the selection process is complete the client may be able to organise and pattern the movements and to make transitions between selected movements.

When mastery such as this is attained, the client will have a movement vocabulary in which to acknowledge, express and communicate within the group, sometimes sharing their dance with the group. Learning the language is part of the process, as in verbal psychotherapy. The dance needs to be repeated and rehearsed to develop or provoke any movement memory. This repetition is a means of exploration and of establishing a personal reality.

Carl Rogers (1967), one of America's most distinguished psychologists, said, 'Learning itself is dependent on wanting to learn, it depends on not knowing the answers but on being willing to explore. It is idiosyncratic and can only significantly influence behaviour if it is self-appropriated learning; truth that has been assimilated in experience.' Movement is experience, and, as with learning, engagement with it is dependent on a willingness to move. Self-understanding is the process of an unfolding adventure common to all learning. As the dance flows into the regressive and out again it offers the freedom for new growth, to rediscover developmental patterns and personal significance in birth, lying, rolling, rocking, kneeling, crawling, standing and walking (*see pp 18 – 26*).

In dance the body is able to re-experience as the sensor, medium and actor, receiving and responding to kinaesthetic, rhythmical and social stimuli. The client becomes aware of their body and its parts, the numerous possibilities for moving in time and space with varying amounts of energy and effort and of moving with their own unique patterns. The process of moving is rewarding for its own sake; **Schilder** (1950) described it as 'loosening up one's body image'.

Structured movement activities based on the clients' own repertoire can lead to improvisation on themes as they emerge. Confidence is gained when movement is repeated and takes place in different contexts, as with a partner or an object. Eventually the client internalises the feeling in the dance and this may become registered at an unconscious level. By making subtle changes in the expressive movement as the group moves together in a group improvisation, the leader reflects the group, yet provides alternatives which may or may not be mirrored by the group.

The process is designed to take the group on a journey from where they are to an extension of that 'here and now'. For example, the movement perseveration (*see Glossary*) of 'rocking' often seen in populations labelled 'autistic' or with severe learning difficulties, may be rediscovered together on the floor, standing or with one person supporting the other. Arms or whole bodies may be rocked, side to side or forward and back. Here the movement is focused upon, although vocalisation and expressive language play an important role with the group who have these possibilities, as does insight. During a mirroring dance in a group or with an individual in the group the leader can gradually make changes in the timing, use of space or effort (*see Laban movement analysis*) and say any words which may express the feeling sense of the movement; some clients, equally, may verbalise or make sounds. This extends repertoire for 'shaping' and 'effort' responses, allowing a wider range of experience in the emotional counterpart to the movement.

The starting-point may come from a theme which developed from a previous session, such as saying goodbye, or it may be something going on at present for the group or individual. It may be exploring a movement theme such as 'opening' or 'closing' or 'jumping'.

A jumping dance might begin with lots of different kinds of jumps. The group can be guided to improvise, then select some favourites or non-favourites to organise and master. Their choice may reflect their mood, their range may be extensive or restrictive; however, it cannot be wrong. To encourage expansion in movement, alternatives are to increase the ability to express moods, attitudes, ideas and behaviours. The jumping dance, once mastered and remembered, may begin to evoke images. These could be explored: for example, fear of falling or always wanting to be up in the sky and never being happy in contact with the ground. Where possible, discussion then makes connections, after which it is important to go back to the movement experience and re-shape it with new consciousness.

It is only when the emotional is worked with in parallel to the physical that change in attitude, self-image and understanding can come about and growth towards full potential can begin. This is the difference between teaching dance and dance movement therapy; the contract is different. Motion and emotion are inextricably intertwined. Movement may be emotionally motivated. The emotion and its intensity evoke the movement; for example, we lunge into assertiveness, squeeze ourselves with delight, stand on our own feet. We are how we move. It is when this is brought into consciousness that changes can take place. The rhythmic nature of dance can bring organisation to what may be a disordered and confused individual or group. Patterns and sequencing of movement and its repetition can help to give the internal locus of control needed by those who are 'acting out'. In addition, non-verbal signals may be more accurately responded to if the client has first been sensitised to their own non-verbal communication and that of others in sessions.

The movement processes themselves are expressive statements in the group, for example, where people place themselves in space in relation to each other and the leader.

In conclusion, however complex the psychopathology of the clients, communication through movement can touch them. We have the same inherent needs and barriers to communication, trust and relationship often found in disturbed or handicapped people. These barriers can be seen in their body boundaries (see Glossary), body image, use of space and movement. They can be overcome by working with their conflicts and motivating their desire for contact and growth, thereby giving them opportunities to form constructive relationships. The pre-verbal, felt and symbolic nature of movement and dance can enable feelings to be identified, explored and expressed, the body, feelings and mind acting as one during the movement.

Work at a verbal and non-verbal level can allow for the felt level to be transformed into body movement through imagery. In those who are able, this precipitates verbal expression at the appropriate developmental level. The reliance on spontaneity and creativity gives a chance for self-directed behaviour and choices and helps release 'frozen', confining behavioural responses and habitual effort patterns (many clients manifest excessive use of one or more of the motion factors, as in, for example, hyperactivity or flaccidity). However it may be necessary to focus on helping the group learn to feel confident in their own spontaneity; or to emphasise learning to play. These new, alternative movement patterns built into the movement vocabulary, with corresponding work with the psychophysical state, can provide the choice of recovery of experiences and can act as a balancing factor for a wider response to the environment.

It is important for anyone using dance movement as a vehicle for growth to be aware of their own movement habits, preferences and psychophysical states in addition to having at their disposal a wide movement repertoire in order to create a non-verbal rapport with the group, using varying qualities, tensions, speeds and so on, enabling other forms of expression and ways of being to emerge.

Effective sessions will depend upon many factors, but specifically upon training and experience in the field of non-stylised dance, group process therapy, and a dance movement therapy training (see Training in Dance Movement Therapy, p 249).

Planning and evaluating a programme

Achievement of physical and emotional integration allows an individual to be more responsive to the environment. Dance and movement activities in a planned programme can help to optimise this integration by:

1 Providing for growth in individual identity; affirmation and the emergence of self through the formation of an adequate body image;

2 Improving social capabilities; developing contact, trust, sensitivity, co-operation with others to enhance decision-making skills and self-confidence;

3 Giving opportunities for expressive use of the body, drawing upon emotional and imaginative resources;

4 Giving a sense of achievement;

5 Generalising movement patterns into a wider variety of situations;

6 Improving functional and dynamic elements of a skill, such as neuromuscular skills in co-ordination of walking;

7 Providing the range of movement needed to allow choice in organising, interpreting and manipulating the world.

Activities involved in your session may or may not be accompanied by music (*see The Use of Music, p 257*). Where music is used you will need to be aware of the 'feeling component' of it. Use it to reflect or contrast with the group feeling. Participants may choose the music or bring in their favourite tapes. These can often act as motivation in the warm-up.

Goals for sessions may be set by the group as a whole, individuals, the staff, the leader or a combination of all these. Goals may be to do with where to go in the group's explorations; group members may even specify the particular behaviour they wish to change, although this does not mean that they are necessarily willing to engage with that change. The 'moving experience' itself may help to uncover goals as well as the realisation of goals. It is important to help clients reflect on their own experience of the session and to aim at small steps, rather than letting them think the sessions will make everything in their lives wonderful. For some groups a pre-treatment interview may be helpful in clarifying what sessions are about and what they feel they could gain. For other groups such an interview may only heighten anxiety levels.

Discussion, feedback and self-disclosure may follow an activity and often connections are made by participants about their experience and realities. It is useful to return again to the movement form, repeating it with this more conscious awareness, noticing what might change and facilitating experimentation with other ways of being.

All sessions need careful thought, and after each session it is crucial to spend time on evaluation, both as a reflection on that session and as a preparation for the planning of the succeeding session.

The development of a session can be seen as a 'creative energy cycle', moving on from the nurturing in the warm-up, to energising in the introduction of the theme, to the climax where the theme is developed in the middle of the session, through to closure where a warm-down finishes the session.

Each stage of the session will vary in length, depending on the phase of development of the group. Warm-ups are generally longer in the early sessions than later on in the group life, but in any event normally do not last more than one-quarter of the total session time. Similarly the warm-down stage should not last more than the final quarter of the session; group members here should be encouraged to leave as individuals separating from the group.

The main work takes place in the middle of the session, where the leader will have selected activities which will help to develop the group themes. These middle stages should take up about half the session time. Introduction of the theme focuses the attention and the development stage involves participants in deeper stimulation.

Ideally the energy cycle should appear as shown in *Figure 1*. This indicates that the group begins and ends with a lower energy level than that found in the middle of a session. Relaxation activities, reflection through verbalisation, integration processes, and awareness focusing on everyday things outside the group can help the transition to closure. You need to ensure that the warm-down finishes in time to close the session punctually. You may need to warn the group that there are only ten, then five, then two minutes left. Always time the activities and let the group know how much time they have at the beginning and have left at the end of each activity.

From the previous session's evaluation it will be evident that a theme has evolved which can be developed in the succeeding session. After deciding upon the overall framework, specific activities which facilitate work on that theme can be planned. However, be prepared for another theme to emerge from the group's warm-up. This may be more relevant to work with at that stage. The leader may choose to reflect the theme or work with its opposite. The linking of themes from session to session gives continuity to the group. In a short time the group will have a life of its own, where particular themes

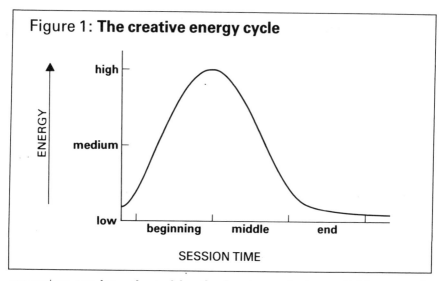

Figure 1: **The creative energy cycle**

ENERGY

high

medium

low

beginning   middle   end

SESSION TIME

emerging can be selected by the leader as being suitable to work with, given the length of time the group will be together, the members' life situations, functioning and anxiety levels. The group responds to the structure provided in a spontaneous, organic manner. The leader will be able to change the structure and activities according to their moods and needs to maintain this spontaneity.

You may find it appropriate, when collecting referrals for your group, to interview each potential participant individually. You may find it helps them to understand the aims and context of the anticipated group and thus be in a position to volunteer to become a participant. Asking them about their expectations of such a group and of movement might also be helpful. Sometimes a written contract can be designed (*see Figure 2 for an example*) and signed by the members. Demonstration sessions are another important aspect of giving an idea to possible participants of what the sessions will be about. Ensure a range of activities are provided for the demonstration session. Expectations need to be verbalised, both from the leader to the group and from the group to the leader.

The first session establishes the initial working relationship with the group as a whole. For those groups with expressive and receptive language abilities, ground rules and the general purpose of the group can be discussed and agreed upon together. This can help engender co-operation and self-responsibility in the group. The ground rules and aims of the group will need to be reviewed regularly and possibly amended. The group and leader need to be clear as to what happens if ground rules are broken.

34

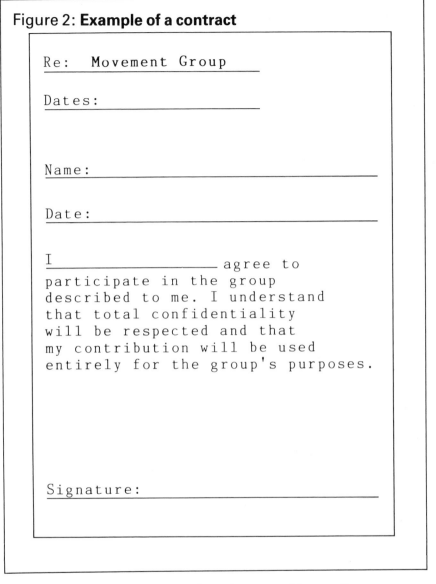

Figure 2: **Example of a contract**

Re: Movement Group

Dates:

Name:

Date:

I _____ agree to
participate in the group
described to me. I understand
that total confidentiality
will be respected and that
my contribution will be used
entirely for the group's purposes.

Signature:

The following ground rules have been used in practice:

1 The session will begin and end on time. All members are
responsible for ensuring this happens (the leader gives times of
sessions and number of sessions for which the group will meet;
any breaks, such as holidays or employment of locums need to be
clarified here).

2   No physical damage to self, others or the environment is permitted.

3   Confidentiality: the content of the group will not be disclosed outside the session unless specifically agreed with the group or individual beforehand.

4   Each member is responsible for their own participation although the leader will encourage all to become involved.

5   No smoking, drinking, eating or chewing gum during the session.

The ground rules, levels of discussion and contract will all depend on the setting, the purpose of the group and the clients' level of functioning. The leader will need to clarify their own personal aims for the group as well as any professional aims. In a team situation, integration of aims already set for clients will need to be incorporated.

It is a good idea to develop a ritual (*see Glossary*) at the start of the session early on in the group life; this may be anything from 'participants removing their shoes' to something more complex which evolves from the group material. Whatever it is, it needs to relax the group and promote anticipation of the session. Rituals to close sessions are sometimes appropriate too.

Early activities in the session can prepare the group for later work; that is, for example, individual breath and vocal work will need to be done if individual moving with the breath and vocalising are to be worked with in depth in the middle stage of the session. Alternatively, if quiet introspection is required for some later partner work, then the warm-up should reflect a quiet atmosphere, with group members in twos.

The approach

There are points of reference which, if taken into consideration, help to involve participants in a creative rhythmic situation more easily than if they were ignored.

The participants will need help to be in touch with their feelings as well as thoughts and to maintain a balance between the two. A carefully chosen structure and direct leadership need to be matched with open-ended spontaneity to facilitate the group's authentic expression.

Since the leader's primary function is to help individuals find an acceptable identity and a more satisfying mode of behaviour for themselves, it is important to maintain a context of flow and focus between both inner and outer processes.

The leader will need to be sincere, offering genuine uncon-ditional acceptance of the group's themes and behaviours and to be empathic with their difficulties. There needs to be an expectancy of success and clear boundaries, including the setting of ground rules at the beginning of a group's life. The 'belief cycle' — where, if the group believes the leader and the leader believes in her methods and medium, the two reinforce one another — creates a positive energy in the group and session as a whole. Eventually the leader should become more of a follower as the group itself takes the lead.

The activities or techniques utilised are only part of the session and should not be viewed as a panacea. No single method is ever effective for all groups, all difficulties or all leaders. It is more important to give attention to the way the activities are used to encourage groups to believe in their own power to help themselves, to acknowledge and solve their own difficulties, to facilitate learning and to mobilise expectancy for success.

It is wise to put theory, method and technique to the back of your mind once you begin the session. It is the process that is in the 'here and now' that needs to be worked with; visualise your feet in contact with the earth to help your own grounding and improve spontaneity and authentic responses, whether they be verbal or non-verbal.

The success will not be in the achievement of a particular movement task or phrase, although spin-offs do lie in the completion of, for example, a stretch jump or a controlled turn into a fall. These are important in the development of confidence in body capabilities and co-ordination, but for growth there needs to be a shift in emphasis from goal-oriented body/movement success to using move-ment and dance as a diagnostic tool and integrating force in the emotional—physical arena.

The leader, in using the activities as a vehicle to reach the group members at their level, may then initiate development to another level (however small the step) so that they may grow in a personal way and any change reverberates through the whole self. By identifying ordinary movement behaviour and crystallising the qual-ities in their movement a recognition of the 'here and now' is brought about, together with the confidence to explore alternative movement as the process evolves towards transpersonal development. There is a balance between the 'here and now' and the 'then and there'.

In dance and movement there is a quality of impermanence which is linked to early stages of play, where the importance lies in doing, not producing. In dance the movement is there and then gone. This may feel safer for some people than methods which formalise and preserve the medium of expression.

Some suggestions for programme structure

1 Having collected your group together you may like to use movement observation (*see p 52*) and/or other observations of behaviour to develop some general aims and identify relevant activities. Base the first session on a variety of activities with the specific objective of assessment. Identify participants' strengths and needs in terms of movement, other non-verbal communication, verbalisation, self-disclosures, participation in the group and so on.

2 When planning the second session you need to build on group strengths rather than limitations, as working with preferred ways to begin with builds self-esteem and can support what may be very weak egos.

3 Ensure that the sessions are at a consistent time and place. You will need to decide whether to 'close' the group to other participants after the first or second session or to leave it as an 'open' group. You will need to be clear with everyone on the number of sessions you will meet for.

4 Use the programme gradually to plan ways in which less preferred ways of moving can be experienced to widen movement resources in the group. Develop variations in the activities to allow for this incorporation, then restructure, redefine and clarify goals for the sessions.

5 Share with others in the setting how the media of movement and dance can help, hinder and provoke changes for the group. Be open to questions, while maintaining confidentiality.

6 Evaluate themes and movement as well as the emotional responses for both individuals and the group as a whole after each session. Reflect on your own style, interventions, feelings and speculations about the session.

7 Develop the resource of movement and dance for use within the treatment programme, specifically in socio-emotional aspects relevant to the organisation.

Anticipated outcomes

As a result of the intervention programme it is hoped that the participants will become more aware and will have internalised several skills and processes in order to fulfil their potential for growth. The following are two possible areas of awareness, with relevant dimensions.

Self-awareness

Sense of internal structure; reduction of impulsivity and perseveration; visualisation skills; imitation skills; self-disclosure; acknowledging and giving others feedback; development of body image, body awareness; wider movement range; isolation and articulation of body parts; adaptability; sensitivity to self; co-ordination skills; assertion skills; decision making.

Social awareness

Co-operation; conforming to a structure; waiting turn; empathy; giving feedback; sharing; leading, following; giving and receiving attention; appropriate physical contact; initiation of activity; group participation; leaving a group and leader.

Forms of evaluation

Evaluation may take place both after each session (formative) and at the end of the programme (summative). It will always need to refer back to the specific goals and general aims. *Figure 3* is an example of a structure for formative evaluation and has been used in practice.

Four sample sessions

The following examples show how a session might be planned for, with overall aims that develop from perceived needs or educational or treatment goals. The session's objectives arise from the previous session, and the theme is introduced and developed in accordance with these objectives. It is important to remember that the activities can be amended to respond to different needs, overall aims and session objectives, and that there are no prescriptive formulae guaranteed to remedy specific difficulties or engender particular responses with any one population.

The following sample sessions are examples of work that has actually taken place; the preliminary session plans have been amended retrospectively to illustrate what actually took place and worked. All the activities have been tried and tested over time; however they will be affected by the style and manner in which they are presented; only you will be able to adapt them to suit your groups and yourself.

The sessions are taken from work in the following settings:

1 Special school (young children);
2 Community home (older children);

Figure 3: **Evaluation sheet for dance movement therapy session**

Date:

Session no:

Present:

Absent:

1 Time and length of session

2 Setting

3 Population

4 Props/music used and reasons

5 Themes predominant (movement and psychodynamic)
a) Themes you arrived with

b) Themes evolving from group

6 What happened overall (including structures used, responses and group dynamics)?

7 Any changes noted?

8 Any specific expressions?
a) Verbal

b) Non-verbal

9 Assessment (include socialisation skills related to objectives; objectives achieved; future objectives for next session).

10 Any other comments?

11 Your own process recording (what happened for you? Include any ideas, images, memories, feelings which emerged for you before, during and after this group session).

Amended from **Payne** (1987)

3 Young people's unit (adolescents);

4 Summer school workshop (adults).

The groups include both verbal and non-verbal clients, with labels such as 'moderate and severe learning difficulties', 'autistic', 'child depressive', 'delinquent', 'school phobic' and 'normal neurotic'.

Example 1: **Special school** *Department of non-communicating children (young children assessed as autistic/psychotic)*

Overall aims
▶ To assess then select four groups, out of 16 children, diagnosing needs, taking into account their overall treatment/educational programme aims.

Session objectives:
▶ To assess the needs of each group member in terms of physical development/capability and relationship.
▶ To assess the helper's role and potential working relationship with each group member; particular attention will be paid to the helper's ease/unease with the movement activities.
▶ To assess members' use of space, awareness of body parts, rhythm, body actions and touch.

Session number 1:
▶ (from a 1-year programme, reviewed intermittently)

Number in group:
▶ Nine, including four helpers — all previously known to each other, having worked together in other treatment programmes. The leader is also well known to all members. This is the first of three groups which are taking part in the initial assessment sessions.

Duration of session:
▶ 45 mins

Gender:
▶ Mixed

Equipment:
▶ Mats
▶ Sticky-backed white tape on floor, making lines.

Warm-up

1   Removing shoes and socks at the edge of the room with help from the helpers, leader says hello to each child and spends some time verbally preparing them for the movement session.

2   Sitting on the white line at the edge of the space, shuffling selves on seats, pushing with hands, over the line, forward and backward as a group. Repeat with rhythmical singing accompaniment: 'We can push ourselves forward, we can push ourselves backward.'

Introduction to theme

1   Each in turn is given a ride by the helper, who stands up to pull the children along the floor on their backs. They move away from the line so that they can still see the group, and then back again. Show helpers how to hold wrists for a firm grip and to use their legs, not backs, to pull. Perhaps sing the child's name and a song saying they are having a ride for each.

2   All at the same time given a pulling ride along floor (corner to corner).

3   In a circle, sitting, hands touching hands, feet, knees, clapping, feet stamping, all to a singing accompaniment.

Development of theme

1   All moving out of circle and into circle on seats, moving in, arriving and clapping, moving out and stamping.

2   Rocking onto backs with feet going high above heads, coming back to centre and clap, clap, clap; again singing accompaniment.

3   Individually, in own space, helper rolls child in a long stretched shape, all crawl back to centre of space.

4   In twos, hand to hand, long rolling together to a corner and running back to centre.

Warm-down

1   Sitting in a partner's lap, enjoy a slow rock, reverse roles.

2   Creeping slowly back to the edge of the space find your shoes and socks and put them on.

3   Leader goes and sits and says goodbye to each person in turn.

What follows is an extract from the leader's notes for this session which may help to illustrate how the session went, what was evaluated, and adjustments decided upon for the succeeding sessions.

When I asked for shoes and socks to be removed this caused some upset for both helpers and children. They were unprepared for this, they expected to work in their shoes, the helpers especially. I need to brief helpers prior to sessions of my expectations and any difficulties they can envisage. I felt very unsure of my ground immediately, I felt this requirement was me forcing my standards upon non-movement orientated people. For the children this was establishing a new routine and one which demanded quite some time to complete. I felt useless only saying hello, so I also helped each helper to remove children's shoes and socks. This made me feel less nervous and framed my 'hellos'.

We sat on the line, all except B who would not, despite lots of encouragement from me and her helper. I felt she was being stubborn; I left her to stand and concentrated on the others, sitting down with them. She seemed very powerful, her tall body overseeing us all. After a minute she joined us sitting. None of them could comprehend directions and all found the floor work difficult, often wanting to stand and run off. It was hard work just to acknowledge their fear and need to escape the containment by separating from the ground and the group. The pushing—slithering was not successful at this stage. The pulling rides were, perhaps because they could feel the physical sensation of the floor in contact with their body more easily as it moved across the floor by an external force, rather than self-initiated. They were able to tolerate touch at this level. The rides from corner to corner were inappropriate — too much space for them to feel secure, too frightening. Perhaps they need to be in a more limited space to concentrate on body awareness through surfaces and rolling action. In future, all floor work needs to involve body awareness and task centred activities (such as moving on hands and knees, elbows and knees, knees only). Contrary to my belief, it seems best not to change the activity too quickly but stick to one for a longer time, modifying it very slightly as it progresses. This was a surprise to me. I thought they would need to change very quickly from one activity to another because of attention spans and interest levels being so limited. Their motor skills, developmentally, were not good but adequate to continue with the floor as their basic support, with a helper. Running was by far the favourite activity — this they nearly all managed very well! Rocking feet over heads was very successful, perhaps the sensation of the rock is exciting, some members are very competent at this on their chairs or on their feet as a ritualized personal movement. Moving in and out of the circle seemed too difficult — not enough boundaries, again lost in space perhaps. More time needed for initial group interactions from the line to the circle formation, possibly leave circle work to the end in future.

Rolling the child was enjoyed by all, but upon my suggestion for the child to roll the helper, although the children were delighted the helpers seemed to feel very vulnerable. They were not used to receiving in this way from the children very often, they may have felt out of control. I will need to bear this in mind when planning the programme. T would not be rolled but did roll his helper, perhaps it appealed to his need to be powerful. Helper J said he would like to be rolled but could not allow it. Something here about letting go of control, being passive to allow self to be rolled. I was also being rolled by a member, which had the disadvantage of my not being in control of the group, not able to hold the space for them; but the advantage of letting helpers and children see me as a model and as able to let go in this way. (Generally, I acted as partner to one of the children.) M very excited, particularly in hand to hand rolling especially when near to the edge of the space, F competent at rolling, rocking and clapping. S seemed afraid to roll onto her front — lots of grimaces of pain. She could only clap once, a soft one, seemed timid throughout session. It felt like she was made of glass, very fragile. There was no synchronous movement or claps/stamps.

Assessment conclusions in relation to some session objectives

1   Brief helpers on movement tasks planned for session.
2   Plan programme around:
    (a)   body parts (hands meeting and parting; knees to chin, etc.);
    (b)   rhythm (singing, claps and stamps to accompany movement with helpers — not in large group);
    (c)   space (task centred to mat/line);
    (d)   body actions (pushing along on seats, rolling);
    (e)   touch (in contact work such as rocking/rolling).
3   Split group into two comprised of: S, M, F,/T and B (able and less able mixed together).
4   Child-helper in a one-to-one relationship (J + S, P + M, R + F, J/L + T).

Overall aims:
▶ The same as the home had identified for each child referred, for example (a) to come to terms with leaving the institution; (b) to reduce anxiety and aggression levels.

Session objectives:
▶ To reduce impulsivity
▶ To work in pairs
▶ To acknowledge their need to compete with each other

Duration of session:
▶ 1 hour

Session number:
▶ 16 (out of a series of 42)

Number in group:
▶ Six

Gender:
▶ Male

Equipment:
▶ Mat per child
▶ Music (tapes)
▶ Drums and other percussion.

Warm-up

Leader counts from one to five and group have to run to touch two walls and return to the centre mat. Who can return first? Leader asks can they now beat their own record. Repeat. Leader asks who they would most like to beat. Repeat activity.

Introduction to theme

1 Leader allocates partners. In turn they follow and move as their partner does, while remaining on their mats (pushed together). Music of one duo's choice is used and the leader turns it off at random, when all have to freeze in stillness for two to three seconds. Movement sections need to be kept short to retain interest. The challenge is for the partner initiating the movement of their choice to make it difficult for their partner to follow. Leader tells the group to change initiators at varied intervals.

2 Leader asks each pair to select a piece of percussion. They use the percussion to accompany their partner's movement for about 30 seconds, when the leader says 'change' and roles are reversed. Partner moving can introduce stillness at any time; the percussionist has to wait until the mover moves again before playing. Challenge is for the mover to try to trick the player into playing while there is stillness. Mats in use to define space.

3 Using all the space the leader drums a beat for all to move to and then freeze when beat stops. Identify the movement activity from members' suggestions, eg. running, leaping etc. At the leader's suggestion each member of the group uses drum for the activity.

4 Leader drums a beat for the group to gather energy and swing into a jump and freeze in a shape, gripping the floor firmly. Two members of group try to move each of the others from their spot, to leader's count of four.

Development of theme

1 In pairs of own choosing, mime any sport. Give two minutes for them to perfect this. Have them slow the mime down considerably, but keeping the same overall pattern. Share each mime, with the others trying to guess the sport portrayed.

2 Leader uses the mime movement as a basis to lead the group in a dance. The group are asked to follow the leader's movement as closely as possible with their own. Each member is on their own mat, while being part of the circle. The leader contrasts the movement with opposite qualities/shapes. Music of their choice is used as an accompaniment (each member gets his choice at some point in the session). If feasible, after bringing the group dance to an end encourage each child in turn to use one of the mime movements to lead the group dance to begin again. After a short time suggest they bring it to an end in stillness.

3 In group discussion encourage each member to remember who they partnered and to say one thing they appreciated about their partner. Have each complete the sentence 'I did not expect . . .' and share it, ask them all how they would describe their behaviour during exercise/whole session.

Warm-down

Lying back on the floor, close eyes and breathe out four times. Tension-release exercise — leader names each body part in turn, beginning with feet and finishing with the face. Open eyes and slowly stand up.

Example 3: **Young people's unit in a Psychiatric Hospital**
(adolescents)

Overall aims:
▶ Same as for their stay in the unit. For example,
  (a) to see if they can become more confident in their body;
  (b) to offer a complementary experience to psychodrama and verbal psychotherapy.

Session objectives:
▶ To reinforce levels of creativity
▶ To be more aware of self in movement and the group
▶ To explore the theme of power in both open and closed body shape.

Orientation:
▶ Non-sexist

Gender:
▶ Mixed

Duration:
▶ 50 minutes

Number in group:
▶ Eight (two staff helpers)

Session number:
▶ Six (in a series of 12)

Equipment:
▶ Music (tapes)
▶ Drum

Warm-up
1 In circle, exercises using stretches forward and side; straightening and bending knees; twisting spine and rising and sinking of whole body. Each repeated four times to music of their choice.

2   In twos, name game using hand gesture to say how they feel today, then repeating saying their name with the same gesture.

3   In circle, whole group repeats name and gesture three times, after each in turn.

4   Leader develops a group movement using the gestures as a basis, exaggerating them and linking them together in a rhythmical pattern. The group move with the leader, following the patterns.

Introduction to theme

In own space; individually close all of the spaces between your body parts and between you and the floor. Make your body feel very closed and tight. Helpers try to 'undo' them, without success. Now make as much space as you can between body parts (can vary the speed with which this is done). Notice the difference; any words to describe this shaping? Standing up, walk across space in your usual manner. Now repeat with tight body shapes and open shapes alternately; which feels familiar to some extent? Discuss in pairs how it felt to do this and to what extent you were aware of your normal shaping.

Development of theme

1   In pairs, A sculpts their partner, B, into the shape they are aware B normally adopts; is it mainly open or wide, or taking up little space? If you do not know, ask B if they are aware. Now exaggerate the shape so that it is more open or closed. Then sculpt them into the opposite shape; ask them for one word which describes how that feels. Go around to look at the other people's shapes, for 30 seconds. Return to partner and tell each other what you experienced, for two minutes. Change roles.

2   With a different partner, sitting back to back, knees up, hands on floor — a competition to push partner across space. Leader beats drum for a short time, they freeze when drumbeat ceases. Now a new partner: one pushes, the other receives the push and guides the direction of travel. Drumbeat. Reverse roles. Discuss how it was to be the pushed and the pusher. Which is the more familiar to you? Give group members a turn on the drum.

3   In the large group, leader asks members: "Select for yourself one person whom you sense is the opposite from the way you feel you are at the moment. In turn say to them why you think that (no response need be made from them). Try to relate it to how you see them sit/stand/move in the unit. It does not matter if you do not

find an opposite, you may like to comment on how you see yourself in terms of body shape." The leader may need to encourage this feedback and to keep the time strictly, eg. spending no more than three minutes.

Warm-down

1 Leader asks for comments on which exercise felt difficult and which felt safe to do. Perhaps ask for them to reflect on what habits have come to their attention today in themselves and others.

2 Return to the shape your partner sculpted you into earlier, move around the room with an awareness of how this feels, taking it up, then moving on alternately.

3 Close eyes and breathe out, noticing the noises outside the room, then those here, especially their own breathing. Slowly, in time with their own breath, open eyes.

Example 4: **Summer school** *as part of summer school workshops (adults)*

Overall aim:
▶ To introduce the use of creative dance for self-awareness and as a process for the self-development of their client groups.

Session objectives:
▶ To create a sense of trust in the group
▶ To aim to overcome some members' inhibitions about movement
▶ To develop group cohesion

Duration of session:
▶ 2 hours

Number in group:
▶ 16

Gender:
▶ Mixed

Session number:
▶ Two (in a series of five)

Equipment:
▶ Music tapes
▶ Parachute

Warm-up

In a circle, each member leads the warm-up, starting with the leader, taking turns spontaneously. They are asked to name a body part they sense as needing to move and to lead the group in a simple movement for that part. Repeat movement eight times to some gentle/lively music of their choosing.

Introduction to theme

1   In pairs, one in front of the other, the first with their eyes closed and forearms up as if the headlights of a car. The one ·behind will guide them by the arms slowly around the space, changing speed, direction, stopping and reversing. Move them as if they are an old car, going uphill, round roundabouts, at traffic lights, turning right and left. Then the leader suggests that they are as if on a motorway, can go faster yet still take good care of their car and avoid others. The leader can direct the tasks as their confidence grows, for five to ten minutes, with a change of roles at intervals.

2   Give a new partner a spin, a ride on your back (need to teach safe support), a lean on you. Change roles. With a new partner again, stand up and sit down together, so sharing your weight with each other sensitively.

3   In threes, trust exercises as in activity 'Relationship 15', p 212.

4   Groups of four or five, as in activity 'Relationship 12', p 210.

5   Groups of six or seven, as in activity 'Relationship 3', p 113.

Development of theme

1   As in activity 'Relationship 12', p 210.

2   Leader presents parachute to the group as a whole, requesting that they unfold it and work with it as a group for 10 minutes. Ask if they would like music; if so, ensure that it is long enough and not overly demanding in energy all of the time. Suggest that they each take it in turn to initiate a movement, beginning with yourself, then name each person, going round the circle. After a while suggest each take a space for themselves to do a special 'trick'. Finally suggest they have one more turn, spontaneously, leading the group, the leader asking for one to lead a closing movement. Perhaps then ask for comments on their experience of the group dance.

Warm-down

As in 'Relationship 13', p 241.

Clients

Some groups require special attention and need placement in rehabilitative, educative or health settings. The reasons are varied. In this text we are concerned with those populations who display behaviour which does not adequately satisfy their needs, and/or is demonstrating a lack of adjustment to the demands of their environment. The labels given to such groups may vary. They include 'at risk', 'emotionally and behaviourally disturbed', 'disaffected', 'socially disadvantaged', 'delinquent', 'personality or conduct disordered', 'problematic', and many are labelled 'psychiatrically disturbed', 'learning disabled' and so on. They may also present with a physical, sensory, linguistic or cognitive handicap.

Having said that, all of us can grow and become more aware if we choose. Humanistic psychology reminds us of this. People do not have to be labelled or in institutions to be in need of opportunities for personal development. This is the reason for including a 'normal' adult group in the sample sessions above. They were attending a workshop as part of a summer school which focused on all the arts therapies: a group which was self-selected, and most were either professionals in one of the helping services or interested artists.

We can, however, make some general assumptions about our clients.

1 A group member's reaction to a space, leader and other participants will, to some extent, be a manifestation of their response in other situations.

2 Every participant is special and can change to extend their potential within the context of the session. Flexibility of response to the emotional and physical demands of life is possible.

3 Opportunities are needed for the individual to learn about themselves in a safe, structured and yet exploratory setting.

4 Dance and movement experiences are one way of re-educating the patterned emotional—physical responses. The purpose is to recover the ability to choose how to live in a positive manner acceptable both to the individual and to society (the implication being that the individual needs to be able to handle society creatively, rather than being pressured into conforming).

5 Movement and dance activities as experiences for growth provide a vehicle for:
   (a) the establishment of individual identity;
   (b) social learning in the opportunities for exploration of generalisable alternative behaviours.

Laban movement analysis

In this material we are concerned with creative movement and dance as means of helping groups with a disturbance and/or disability to organise and develop a repertoire of behaviour which will enable them to satisfy their own needs and adjust more adequately to the demands of their environment. Since we are working at a body—movement level as well as an emotional and learning level a system of language which can help identify and clarify movement themes, movement objectives and observations is important.

Laban's contributions were both in the promoting of creative dance and in his system for observing and categorising movement. In this system attention is shifted towards the vocabulary, analysis and observation of movement; what we move (body), how we move (effort), where we move (space) and with what or whom we move (relationship).

By observing through these categories we become sensitised to the range of movement behaviour people have, their strengths and limitations expressed as 'effort habits' and 'shaping preferences'. From this information (and an assessment of behavioural aspects as gained through tests, observation charts and checklists) a programme of dance and movement sessions relevant to the person's needs can be developed.

Laban viewed movement holistically, as a process — the fragments of body, effort, space and relationships added together do not make the whole, the whole is greater than the parts which are combined together. Movement is only a part of behaviour, but in observing and describing or defining it we can be aware of the variation within that behaviour. The reintegrative process can be helped without verbal acknowledgement by client or therapist, through gradual or sudden changes in the movement. However it must not be a prescriptive or 'filling in the gaps' approach, such as might be found in rote learning or imposed dance exercises which are isolated from the total organism. These are 'conditioned' responses and are not spontaneous or authentic in the multi-level process.

There is no need for psychological training to decode messages communicated non-verbally (eg. a depressed posture), nor is specific training needed to be aware of a person's physical presence, which could be strengthened by moving experiences in re-education. Sensitivity as a mover, leader and observer are required, however, and courses may help to heighten this awareness (*see section 4, Training in Dance Movement Therapy*). There are cross-cultural variants which need to be contextualised, for example when working with multi-ethnic groups (**Blacking**, 1977).

Movement observation is valuable in three ways:

1 as a tool for identifying the individual movement strengths and limitations. Movement observations are only a starting-point and should be pooled with other information before assessing the needs and developing a relevant programme;

2 as a device that enables you to observe the client outside the confines of other relationships;

3 as a method of identifying movement themes and the setting of movement goals for the group within the session.

Laban Movement Analysis may be summarised as follows:

What moves

This is the 'body' as a whole, its different parts in isolation and in co-ordination.

Shapes in movement or stillness

(a) curled

(b) stretched

(c) wide

(d) twisted
(*See Glossary.*)

Activity
Locomotion, elevation, turns, gestures, stepping, stillness.

Body Parts
Knees, arms, hands, head etc.

Symmetry
Both sides of the body doing the same thing simultaneously.
(*See Glossary.*)

Asymmetry
One side of the body moving independently and/or differently from the other.

Body Flow
Successive or simultaneous; peripheral or central. Body parts initiating/leading movement.

How the body moves

This is the quality of the movement termed 'effort', comprised of combination of factors (dynamics and textures) conveying our inner attitudes thoughts and feelings. There are four main factors:

Time
Revealed through suddenness (sharp, quick, urgent) and sustainment (prolonged, unhurried, slow).

Weight
Revealed by the degree of muscular tension varying between firm (forceful, resistant, strong) and light (delicate, gentle, buoyant).

Space
Identifies the extent to which a movement is generous or economic in the use of space — it may be between extremes of directness (undeviating, straight) and flexibility (indirect, roundabout). This is not to be confused with *where the body moves*.

Flow
This factor concerns the freedom of flow or restraint with which a movement is carried out, the extremes being free, fluent, easy and ongoing movement that can only be stopped with difficulty, and tightly controlled, bound, restricted movement that can easily be stopped at any point in its journey.
NB. It is a combination of these 'efforts' which makes vehicles for our feelings.

Where the body moves — space

Personal space
This is the space into which we move, immediately surrounding the body. *Inner space* That which is contained inside our bodies.

General space
That which is outside the immediate reach, where we find ourselves,

eg. corridor/ward/hall/playground. We move into general space taking our personal space with us.

Levels
High, medium and low. Movement takes place at any of these levels and in different directions.
(*See Glossary.*)

Directions
Forward, backward, to one side and the other, upwards and downwards and all the way around. *Diagonals* are a combination of these.
(*See Glossary.*)

Extension into space
Near or far.

Air and floor pathways
Curved/straight patterns can be carved out of the air and on the floor with gestures or whole body.
(*See Glossary.*)

Space Actions
Rise—sink/open—close/advance—retreat.

With whom or what we move — relationship (*See Glossary*)

Relatedness of body parts to each other, relationship to self.
Relationship of individuals to each other.
Relationship of groups to each other.
Relationship to environment: objects, space.

Relationship implies the world of people, objects and stimuli with whom and with which we live, work and play. It implies listening, watching, initiating or responding to contact. *Body* (what), *effort* (how) and *space* (where) all hinge upon the core issue of *relationship*, without which growth would not take place.

By extracting the major areas of Laban Movement Analysis a number of possible starting-points can be illustrated diagrammatically. (*See Figure 4.*) The idea is that each area is connected, yet grows out of the whole. The emphasis of the experience offered may only be in one area, however. The figure gives an overall picture of the way each aspect can be viewed as interrelated, layer upon layer. Supplementary aspects have been included where they are thought to be particularly relevant to groupwork, for example 'Breathing', 'Rhythm' 'Body Boundaries' (*see Glossary*) and 'Pre-laterality'.

Figure 4

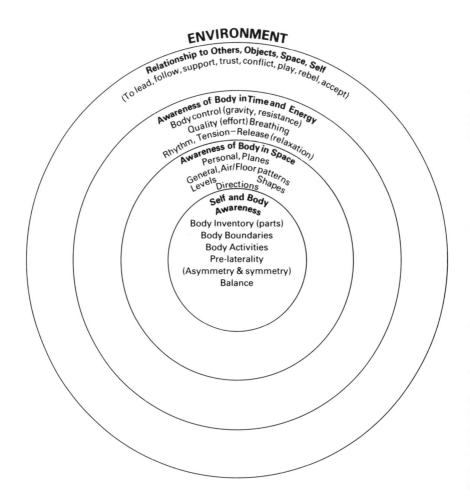

ENVIRONMENT
Relationship to Others, Objects, Space, Self
(To lead, follow, support, trust, conflict, play, rebel, accept)

Awareness of Body in Time and Energy
Body control (gravity, resistance)
Quality (effort) Breathing
Rhythm, Tension–Release (relaxation)

Awareness of Body in Space
Personal, Planes
General, Air/Floor patterns
Levels   Shapes
Directions

Self and Body Awareness
Body Inventory (parts)
Body Boundaries
Body Activities
Pre-laterality
(Asymmetry & symmetry)
Balance

Guidelines for group leaders

Personal preparation for session

The following points may be useful to you, particularly when working with very difficult groups.

1   Rehearse and visualise where, with whom, and how the session will take place.

2   Look at your apprehensions/fears for the sessions, for example your feelings about your own body and movement and acceptance of the work with colleagues. How will you overcome these?

3   What do you expect to go well in the session?

4   What will be the most difficult problem? What strategy will you use to overcome it?

5   Decide on the minimum response from the group that you will be satisfied with.

6   What do you think the group needs as a minimum response to feel satisfied?

7   Read through your evaluation notes from the previous session and plan for this one.

8   Put the plan to the back of your mind so that you can be open to responses from within the group. Be prepared to mould your plan around relevant themes emerging.

9   Think about what equipment you require, and its collection. Can it be used safely in the space? When will you use it?

10 How will you finish?

11 Immediately prior to the session, centre yourself in a quiet place, alone.

Hints on the environment

A structured, safe environment gives an opportunity to participate in the movement dialogue with the leader or others, using latent and manifest sources of movement symbolism to understand and recognise how they conduct their life and how they can alter it.

It may be best to start with a small space: a classroom, music room, meeting place, etc. You need to be sure that this can be used exclusively by your group during the session time; interruptions can be very disturbing to any groupwork. You may need to be prepared for clients to have some associations with the space prior to your session, for example as a place for talking, playing, being quiet, doing schoolwork, being in another type of group or activity.

Some noise may be made in your group, so you may need to find out if this would cause anyone else outside the session inconvenience and, if so, to negotiate for a relocation and so on.

A large gymnasium or hall may prove threatening and overwhelming to your group. If this is the only space available, try sectioning it off with benches, tables and mats.

Be aware of any distractions in the space (eg. mobiles, mirrors, pictures, books, instruments). Remove these whenever possible and ensure that the space remains consistent over time, both in its internal decoration and in its availability, to promote added security for the groups.

You need to keep the space sparsely furnished and the floor clean. Carpets tend to be an inhibition to movement and nylon carpets are positively dangerous. Small mats, cushions or chairs could be used for the beginning or end of the session, if felt appropriate, to focus the group. For some populations, for example those with a physical handicap, the elderly or long-stay psychiatric, chairs may need to be kept as their base throughout the session, especially at first. Certainly for discussion times cushions are often more comfortable for some groups. Mats are ideal for discussions and other activities you may wish to try. Small and light gym mats or yoga/exercise mats are best.

Encourage the group to remove shoes and socks at the start of each session, and insist on loose clothing. Have a cassette player (not batteries) nearby for use and encourage participants to bring in tapes they like to move to.

Working with colleagues

When working with other staff in the group you need to ensure that you have negotiated expectations with each other. For the physically less able, sensitive and supportive help from other members of your team (eg. a physiotherapist) may be useful. It is invaluable to have evaluation and planning communications between numerous different colleagues. In this way the programme may be designed from shared information in the interest of all group members and which is congruent with the establishment's overall aims/rehabilitation programme. You need to be prepared to translate your work into a vocabulary colleagues can understand.

Guidelines for sessional practitioners attempting an intervention programme of DMT
(adapted from material first published in Payne, 1988)

While the following may seem obvious, they appear as guidelines; they can be disregarded or disagreed with, especially if you feel intuitively that they are not a good idea for your clients or yourself in your setting.

1 You will need to be clear about your aims and objectives and how you plan to implement them.

2   Spend time liaising with the principal or director of the establish-ment and the educational/clinical psychologist first, explaining the project and eliciting their prejudices/biases, if any.

3   You may wish to give a presentation to all staff, outlining the project and focusing on the need for their full co-operation and support. Do not promise or guarantee anything; there is a tenden-cy for staff to believe that the 'outsider' holds a magic formula and will change 'bad' behaviour into 'good' overnight. Explain any benefits that have taken place, however, as a result of previous programmes.

4   It may be desirable to give a demonstration session to the potential clients and staff. As a result of this, volunteers may come forward, willing to participate in the project. Limit numbers to between four and eight per group, although the numbers will be dependent on levels of functioning.

5   You will need to be careful about what you tell the clients and staff about the sessions — the words you use and the information you give will be determining factors in the attitude they will present about sessions. For example, with male adolescents labelled 'delinquent' the sessions may be called 'movement' rather than 'dance', which could avoid stereotypes in their minds and those of the staff.

6   You need to be aware of the institutional philosophy, time management, organisational resistance and so on. You may need to adapt your programme to fit in with this in order to avoid conflict and confusion for staff and clients.

Support groups

Many of the enquiries received by the Association for Dance Movement Therapy (ADMT) (*see section 4 for address*) come from people interested in beginning work in the field or already quietly involving themselves in using dance and movement in establishments with various populations all over the UK. There seems to be an overwhelming need for contact with others who are working in a similar way.

In addition, people seem to need reassurance that what they are doing with their groups or individuals is 'OK': that is, it can be understood and has some value in its own right. They also need contact and support, an opportunity to share work difficulties and to consult with others — outside their work setting — about their groups and sessions.

The ADMT came into being to meet just such a need (**Payne** 1983). A small group of individuals met regularly in London to discuss their work, to tease out theoretical issues as they arose, and above all to 'move' together. This support group, as it was now termed, met for several years and gradually grew into what is now known formally as the ADMT. This, however, was the spin-off; the underlying desire was that need for support.

The support group can be seen to have four main objectives:

1 To make and maintain contact with others involved in, and sympathetic to, the use of dance and movement in groupwork;

2 To gain support for each other in what may be a vague and unknown area — and to work creatively together to overcome some of the difficulties in the work;

3 To explore other ideas in order to be useful to patients/clients: the support group is often a safe place to try out these ideas;

4 To create dancing experiences for each other and relate these to groupwork.

Guidelines for your support group meeting

If you wish to form or be part of a support group the following are points which may be used, changed or rejected as you see fit. All groups are different and these guidelines may offer a springboard for some of them.

1 Ensure that you have each other's names, addresses and telephone numbers.

2 Take it in turns to be the 'contact person' to arrange suitable days/times for meetings and to book the space.

3 If possible, meet centrally and in the same place. Church halls, drama halls, dance studios, colleges or schools may be suitable.

4 How often do you wish to meet? (This will depend on commitment, cost, place, group dynamics and so on.)

5 Do you wish to liaise with ADMT to gain members? (*See Useful Addresses*). How large or small do you want the group to be? (Five to six members is often appropriate.)

6 What is the function of your group? What do you expect, what can you contribute, what are your hidden desires? How are you going to review the purpose of the group and its work?

7 Do you want to take it in turns to lead the group, experimenting with different activities and receiving feedback?

8   What topics do you wish to consider? These might include how to activate and motivate groups, transference, resistance, touch, verbalisation, sexuality, creativity, use of video, sound and props, leaving a group.

9   Allow space for members to bring difficulties, finding a way to work with them as in role-play, or dancing out an issue based on a theme. One or two members may wish to watch, to give feedback on their perceptions of the process.

10   Are you going to share information gained from participation in relevant courses or workshops, reading lists, or have a loan system for articles or books?

11   Do you wish to visit each other's working environments? This may promote greater understanding of the context in which support group members work.

12   Make notes for yourself after each meeting.

13   What restrictions are there in your work? Can the group help you find creative ways of overcoming these?

14   Do you want to bring in outside leaders?
      Remember that groups have their own dynamics. Stay with the work of the group, rather than exploring the dynamics of the group — that is, unless they really shout at you!

Supervision

The question of supervision often does not arise at the beginning of group leaders' paths into this field. You may have colleagues or others to consult over issues, despite limitations of experience. However, the importance of supervision from experienced practitioners from outside any support group or work setting is vital.

In the UK, unfortunately, there are only a limited number of experienced leaders in the field able to offer supervision. If there is not one in your area, there may be a skilled therapist who might be encouraged to offer you supervision on a regular basis — preferably an arts therapist or a psychotherapist. Some of the problems arising in groupwork and therapy are universal: for example, finishing a programme of work, over-involvement and so on. These may all be issues you could discuss in relation to your own population. Any good therapist — whatever their school or approach — may be helpful for supervision (*see section 4 for some useful addresses*).

Personal therapy

Concerning your own personal therapy, this is often the last to be considered for attention! We are frequently quick and ready to offer ourselves as therapists, without having undergone any therapy or groupwork ourselves.

Long-term intensive group or individual therapy is as important as professional training and supervision for anyone intending to work or already working in DMT. Ideally, a dance movement therapy group itself would fit the bill. However, since DMT practitioners are scarce in the UK, in a freelance capacity, one of the arts therapies, Group Analytic, Gestalt, Psychodrama and other group approaches would serve. One-to-one therapies, including Reichian, Transactional Analysis, Psychosynthesis or individual psychoanalysis (Jungian/Freudian) may be alternatives. However, if you intend to work with groups it is advisable to have had a group experience. It is very important to be discerning when selecting a therapy and a therapist. Be clear about what you want, and feel good about the therapist you have selected. (*See section 4 for some useful addresses.* Please note that their inclusion is not to be perceived as recommendation.)

What is the role of the dance/movement worker in relation to the dance movement therapist?

This issue needs to be addressed when many group leaders are working in the field without a formal training in dance movement therapy. The following may help clarify some of the issues. The Standing Committee for Arts Therapies Professions has published a document to help employers and others to be more aware of this sometimes confusing issue (*see section 4, p 253 and footnote below*).

The dance/movement worker, who may have training in teaching, dance, occupational therapy, group work or another related area, has a complementary role to that of the dance movement therapist. Both work with individuals of all ages who have social, emotional, sensory, cognitive and physical problems (some of these problems are present together). Both are employed to work with individuals and groups by agencies such as psychiatric hospitals, clinics, day care services, community health centres, special schools

---

A leaflet entitled *Artists and Arts Therapists — their Roles* sets out more details on this topic. It is available from Hertfordshire College of Art & Design, 7 Hatfield Rd, St Albans, Herts. Cost: £2.00.

or prisons. Both can act as consultants and may engage in research, and both need to identify their overall aims for their groups, whether creative, educational or therapeutic.

Experience of working with special needs groups in dance and movement is valuable for those wishing to train as dance movement therapists.

The dance/movement worker

Practitioners such as qualified physical educators, dance teachers or dance artists aim to give opportunities in the media of dance and movement to special needs groups, who would otherwise normally be excluded from such experiences. The relationship is teacher to student, rather than therapist to client, and the contract is different from therapy: the emphasis is on enjoyment, aesthetic pleasure and education, such as knowledge and understanding of and skills in dance and/or movement. The experiences on offer may include visits to dance performances; undertaking a series of classes with a dance company, leading to a final performance in the establishment; and workshops with a group and their teachers, which again may help a group to perform dances in the hospital or school and so on. Workers may also include groups of people with a disability as equal partners in classes and as dance performers.

Through such experiences the senses may be heightened and a potential discovered. Physical and perceptual skills may be fostered, and areas such as body awareness, self-image, intuition and the integration of thought and emotions may be enhanced. These are all important spin-offs, but the modification of symptoms and/or engagement with the emotional life of the client is not the primary purpose for this type of practitioner. Rather, they seek to develop opportunities for educating and enriching lives and to create positive achievements. Their aim is to offer dance as an art form, and performance (not necessarily public) is often an outcome of their work.

The dance movement therapist

The major role of this practitioner is to complement that of the dance/movement worker. She aims to bring about, with someone whose development has been arrested or has taken an abnormal path, durable, positive change in the direction of physical, emotional and social well-being, or to help a person more fully achieve their potential.

The dance or movement activity and any resulting formed dance becomes the method for diagnosis and further therapeutic intervention, or a vehicle for supporting the health of the client. The dance movement therapist, educated in both the human sciences and dance/movement forms, is committed to the therapeutic use of dance and movement as a discipline to further the person's emotional growth and psychological and social integration. They select from their wide-ranging therapy, dance, movement and observation skills to enable contact with otherwise isolated and difficult client groups. They work in treatment, rehabilitative and special educational settings. They plan and evaluate sessions and work towards agreed therapeutic goals, often within a multidisciplinary team. Sometimes this practice takes place as a prerequisite for those clients unable to benefit from the dance worker's input, or alongside their work. In common with the other arts therapies, an important dimension of dance movement therapy is that it offers simultaneous access to both feeling and symbolic levels of human experience.

Professional dance movement therapists have a training which includes a range of dance and movement skills, core therapy skills, clinical studies, anatomy and physiology, anthropology, human development, observation of movement, and research, assessment and evaluation skills. They are regularly supervised for practice and have experienced their own therapy.

These two types of practitioner are therefore not mutually exclusive; they do, however, have different priorities and, in consequence, training needs to acknowledge these differences.

Conclusion

This section has covered the main theoretical aspects, including developmental movement processes, non-verbal communication, the facilitation of expressive dance and suggestions on the planning and evaluation of programmes. Four sample sessions served to illustrate some of the issues referred to in the text. Laban Movement Analysis was presented for reference and some guidelines were suggested which may aid those new to the field in gaining some support for their work. Finally, the roles of worker and therapist were briefly explored.

Helping clients to grow towards more healthy functioning through the use of creative dance and movement requires an approach which makes use of action and reflection. Through the use of movement observation skills to assess the type of intervention required, and the adaptation of a planned programme of work according to the changing needs of the group, participants will be able to engage with themes appropriate to their psychophysical stages of development. There needs to be a clear contract with the group and work setting which states whether the programme is therapy or not. Those using the media of creative movement and dance need to be aware of the roles of worker and therapist and to develop their own guidelines and support for setting up programmes of work.

ACTIVITIES

INTRODUCTION

What follows is a sample of ideas for activities which have proved useful in practice. They will need to be adapted to be made suitable for your group and yourself. It is important to view them as a starting-point and to integrate them as part of the overall programme which the clients are involved with, whether it be educational or rehabilitative in focus. The activities presented here will therefore need to be amended to relate to clients: specifically to their intellectual, spiritual, physical and emotional developmental levels. They should not be used 'cold', as isolated exercises, as 'a fill-in', but as part of a pre-planned and integrated approach.

It is wise to begin with the activity you feel most comfortable with; normally you will need to have experienced it yourself and to have practised or rehearsed it, in your support group perhaps.

The activities are divided into four sections:

Warm-up: which may be useful in the initial stages of a session;

Introduction to theme: which sets the scene for a particular movement idea or could reflect a group theme;

Development of theme: which is a more in-depth activity to take the group further into a particular idea;

Warm-down: for use in closing sessions.

Guidelines for physical safety

1   You will need to have some basic knowledge of how the body functions anatomically and physiologically before attempting to use movement with client groups (*see section 4 for institutions offering relevant courses*).

2   Before embarking on a programme you will need to be aware of any group member who (a) presents a medical problem or (b) is on medication; either may affect their level of participation. This may require access to client files and discussion with the person responsible for the client; it may also require the negotiation of confidentiality before any such material is made available to you as group leader.

3   For all groups you will need to be aware of participants' physical limitations (eg. heart problems).

CRAB FOOTBALL

Aims: To warm up group physically, release energy

Population: Children/adolescents

Conditions: Early sessions; no violence

Time: 10 minutes

Equipment: Soft medium-size ball, goals (wide goal for less skilled group); playing area appropriate for fitness level of group

Structure: Two equal groups

■Activity

1 Two teams identified and shooting ends given.
2 Everyone on all fours, stomachs uppermost; only pass or shoot with feet.
3 Play for 4–5 minutes each way.

■Supplementary development of activity

1 Must make four passes before shooting.
2 Change size of playing area.

■Additional outcomes

Competition, accepting boundaries, working as a group.

BODY SENSATION 1

Aim: To experience body sensations through movement
Population: All
Conditions: Safety element, regular stops to re-orientate
Time: 5 minutes
Equipment: None
Structure: Individual, pairs

■Activity

1   Spin on the spot, feeling the air rushing past.
2   Spin with a partner; use a firm handgrip (eg. wrist to wrist).
3   Notice how your body feels afterwards.

■Supplementary development of activity

1   Swing arm through air.
2   Swing leg.
3   Walk, to jog, to sprint.

■Additional outcomes

People become aware of the sensations in their body as they move quickly through the space. They become more in touch with their bodies through these exercises.

BODY SENSATION 2

Aims: To become more aware of the tensions in our bodies; to begin to release tension

Population: All

Conditions: None

Time: 5 minutes

Equipment: Drum

Structure: Individual

■Activity

1 While lying on the floor in open position, let eyes close.
2 Leader talks through a count of 1 to 5, during which each member tenses their whole body, including face, and holds breath.
3 Count down from 5 to 1 and release tension built up.
4 Count down from 5 to 1 again for further release, using breath.
5 Repeat the above for specific body parts identified by group member.

■Supplementary development of activity

1 Use drum for build-up of tension; build up slowly in a crescendo.
2 Tension could be expressed in contraction, extension or twisting of body.

■Additional outcomes

Sense of the tension required and of excessive habitual tension which needs release. Quiet time can enable deep awareness of body.

See page 237 for this activity used in another stage.

BALANCE 1

Aims: To develop self-control and body awareness
Population: All
Conditions: None
Time: 4–5 minutes
Equipment: Music if desired
Structure: Individually and large group

■Activity

1 On spot in circle, move one isolated body part (for example, circling an arm). Leader begins by modelling movement.
2 After a few of these, give opportunity for participants to identify and articulate one body part in turn around the group. Say out loud the name of the body part and the type of articulation.

■Supplementary development of activity

1 Move two body parts.
2 Move one body part while the rest of the body is in a specified shape, eg. kneeling, sitting, legs astride.

■Additional outcomes

1 Awareness in large group; turn-taking and following in rhythmic pattern.
2 Identification and articulation of body parts.

See page 107 for this activity used in another stage.

BALANCE 2

Aims: To develop control of body; to break 'rules'

Population: Children, adolescents, 'acting-out' adults

Conditions: Early sessions

Time: 5 minutes

Equipment: Drum

Structure: Individual

■Activity

1 Group at one side of room.

2 Walk across room and stop very still when hear drum, which beats rhythmically. Aim is to continue walking when feel like it, while drum still playing. Since the overt 'rule' is to 'stay still until the drum stops', they must aim to break that rule. Leader to ensure they understand that the rule can be broken.

3 Hold stillness while drum continues.

4 Ask for volunteer to drum. They can make a guess at who will break the rule each time.

■Supplementary development of activity

1 Repeat, but run across room.

2 Repeat, but slide on belly across room.

3 Leader turns back on the group while drumming, so cannot see group.

■Additional outcome

Acknowledgement that 'rule-breaking' is possible in this structure.

See page 110 for this activity used in another stage.

LOCOMOTION 1

Aims: To move in accordance with a set rhythm, travelling (*see Glossary*) in a co-ordinated, rhythmic experience

Population: Children, adults

Conditions: None

Time: 10 minutes

Equipment: Drum, music of your choice

Structure: Whole group as individuals, in partners, trios

■Activity

1 Leader beats out a rhythm on the drum or puts on the music.
2 Leader varies the rhythm and calls out ways of travelling (eg. walk, gallop, slide, jump, slither).

■Supplementary development of activity

1 Join up with a partner and follow the pattern of travelling the partner selects, while leader continues to beat out a rhythm; then repeat, reversing roles.
2 Repeat in trios, small groups, periodically changing the person deciding the pattern.
3 Let a volunteer beat out rhythm on drum or select the music for the group.

■Additional outcomes

1 More trust develops as the leader is accepted.
2 All members can initiate their own ideas for travelling within the safety of a clear rhythmic pattern.
3 The group learns to follow the lead from others and turn-taking is experienced in taking the lead.

See page 157 for this activity used in another stage.

LOCOMOTION 2

Aim: To promote movement range in locomotion (*see Glossary*)
Population: All
Conditions: None
Time: 5–10 minutes
Equipment: Plentiful space
Structure: Whole group

■Activity

1 Leader suggests group walk at normal pace around room, individuals changing directions at will.
2 Speed up walk to become a jog.
3 Speed up jog to become a run.
4 Slow down run to regain the jog.
5 Slow down jog to return to walk.
6 Slow down walk to become twice as slow.
7 Twice as slow again.
8 Twice as slow. Ensure in this final stage that the movement is very sustained, ie feet moving through the stages of walking and participants concentrating on the minute movement from one stage to the next as transfer of weight etc takes place.

■Supplementary development of activity

Repeat above, beginning with slow walk and increasing run, then sprinting.

LOCOMOTION 3

Aims: To accept outside structure, co-ordination, rhythmic experience

Population: Children, adults

Conditions: None

Time: 10 minutes

Equipment: Drum, music of your choice

Structure: Whole group as individuals, in pairs, threes

■Activity

1 Leader beats out a rhythm on the drum or puts on the music.
2 The group move at a walk, gallop, slide, jump, slither (etc) as instructed by the leader.

■Supplementary development of activity

1 Can join up with a partner and follow in the pattern of locomotion partner selects, then reverse roles.
2 Repeat in threes, small groups.
3 A volunteer beats out the rhythm and/or selects the music.

■Additional outcomes

More trust develops as the leader is accepted. All members can initiate their ideas for locomotion within a clear rhythmic pattern. Following and turn-taking are experienced.

BODY BOUNDARY 1

Aim: Awareness of physical boundaries
Population: Children
Conditions: First sessions
Time: 5 minutes
Equipment: None
Structure: Individual

■Activity

On leader's signal all run to a specified part of the room and push against it (eg. wall, centre of floor) using hands and arms for the count of five. Use all strength, wide base (ie legs apart, one leg in front of the other and knees bent if standing) grit teeth etc.

■Supplementary development of activity

1   Push with backs or sides.
2   Push for a longer count.
3   Run and touch three or four places on the edge of the space and return to the centre within the count of five.

■Additional outcomes

Knowledge of the physical space. Energy is built up for session.

NAMEGAME 1

Aim: To learn names
Population: All
Conditions: None
Time: 10 minutes
Equipment: None
Structure: Group and pairs

■Activity

1 Each says own name in turn around the circle.
2 Each says own name and adds an accompanying gesture.
3 Repeat (2) above; after each person's contribution the group echo the name and gesture three times.

■Supplementary development of activity

1 Go away and, individually, select 2 or 3 [leader stipulates] movements you liked doing from the previous group activity. Link them up. This is a sentence of movement — rehearse it.
2 Join with a partner and move your sentence. Partner has to guess the 2 or 3 names these movements were linked to.
3 Join up partner's movements and own to form a longer sentence.
4 Make the sentence of movement travel across the space.
5 Add sounds (eg. the names) to the movement.
6 Share with another twosome.

■Additional outcomes

1 Linking movements together.
2 Performing a movement phrase for others.

NAMEGAME 2

Aim: To ground group in the present
Population: All
Conditions: Early in programme (first session)
Time: 10 minutes
Equipment: None
Structure: Whole group

■Activity

1 In a group circle, say your name in turn around the circle.
2 Next say your name and one 'thing' you notice.
3 Next say your name and express in movement that noticed 'thing'.
4 Whole group then mirror back the movement made once.

■Supplementary development of activity

Leader uses all their movements (and group echoes). Leader initiates and develops them to link together with accompanying music.

■Additional outcome

Recognise and learn the names of people in group.

NAMEGAME 3 (Silly Walks)

Aims: To promote travelling movement activity and creativity;   to learn each other's names

Population: Adults

Conditions: First session

Time: 20 minutes

Equipment: None

Structure: Partners/whole group

■Activity

1   Find a partner, exchange names and invent three different silly ways of walking. Share ideas with a partner.

2   With the same partner, stand opposite, say their name, and use one of the walks to change places. Repeat this, each using all three walks. (Start 5 or 6 feet apart, no physical contact.)

3   Find a new partner, exchange names. Repeat stage 2, using the favourite walk so far.

4   Find another partner, exchange names. Repeat stage 2, using the least favourite walk.

5   Find a final partner, exchange names. Repeat stage 2, using the walk you have left out so far. Can you remember the names of the last three partners?

■Supplementary development of activity

1   Make a large group circle, place yourself opposite your original partner. Check that you know their name.

2   Spontaneously, but in turns, say your partner's name and exchange places, using one of your walks.

3   Repeat this several times, so that all partners have exchanged places. The rest of the group is to notice the names as they are shouted out, as well as the way people walk.

4   When you think you know another person's name, shout that name out; they then have to change places with you. Each person is to use one of the invented silly walks from the original three.

■Additional outcomes

The whole group will be able to recall and say at least three names from the group, and everybody's name if the development has been used; they will often remember people by their walks.

SHAKING OUT

Aim: To identify physical sensations in body

Population: Children, adolescents, adults

Conditions: Any session

Time: 5–10 minutes

Equipment: None

Structure: Whole group, partners

■Activity

1   Whole group in circle. Leader suggests they all shake out different body parts in turn. Can use similes, eg. 'shaking off drops of water'. Always go from periphery towards centre of body, eg. hand, lower arm to upper arm. Leader models.

2   After first part has been thoroughly shaken out, stop and ask participants to compare any sensations with those in parts not yet moved.

3   Allow people to mention any aspects that they notice in their own bodies, eg. tingling or warmth in the energised arm, numbness in the non-activated arm.

4   Work through the whole body systematically. Could sing an accompaniment to the exercise if appropriate.

■Supplementary development of activity

Partners shake out some body parts, eg. feet, legs.

■Additional outcomes

1   The participants become aware of own bodies and their physical sensations.

2   Focus is on the body — sets the scene for rest of session.

BODY CONTROL 1

Aims: To reduce impulsivity and perseveration
Population: Children
Conditions: None
Time: 3 minutes
Equipment: Drum
Structure: Individual

■Activity

1   Suggest the group move very quickly all over the space to drumming.
2   When drum stops they freeze and hold position.
3   Repeat freezing in different position each time.

■Supplementary development of activity

1   Use drum as signal to stop — ie when drum is banged, freeze.
2   Have volunteer play drum.

■Additional outcome

Offers opportunity to control body from movement to stillness.

BODY CONTROL 2

Aim: Introduce idea of assertion in body shape and energy

Population: All

Conditions: Warmed-up joints

Time: 2 minutes

Equipment: Drum

Structure: Individual

■Activity

1 Using a drum as accompaniment, leader suggests participants run and jump and finish in a strong shape — tall, wide, twisted, angular, rounded.

2 Select someone to help you to attempt to push the members to see how strongly they can hold their shape.

3 Ensure that the group use wide bases and bend at the knees in their shapes to resist the attempts at pushing them over by the volunteer.

4 Repeat with the suggestion of a different shape each time.

■Supplementary development of activity

1 Extend the above by adding:

 (a) a half-fall,

 (b) a turn,

 (c) ·a movement,

 after the shaping in stillness.

2 Volunteer could accompany with a drum.

■Additional outcome

Phrasing and combining movement forms.

FLOOR PATTERN 1

Aim: To develop adaptability on moving across the floor

Population: All

Conditions: None

Time: 3–4 minutes

Equipment: Lively, rhythmical music

Structure: Individual, partner

■Activity

1   Explore patterns and shapes across floor using feet to step them out (participants can choose their own patterns and shapes or leader can give examples).

2   Each make up a step pattern which carves out a shape on the floor.

3   Repeat, but using music to accompany patterning.

4   Repeat the pattern, making the movement smaller/larger, covering whole of the floor space.

■Supplementary development of activity

1   Follow a partner's step pattern and repeat.

2   Teach pattern to partner and step out together both patterns.

FLOOR PATTERN 2

Aim: To experience leading and following as a linked group

Population: Adults, children (adolescents if stick or material used instead of hand-holding)

Conditions: None

Time: 3–4 minutes

Equipment: None

Structure: Whole group

■Activity

1 The group make a line, holding hands. Designate one of the people on the end as leader.

2 For one minute they walk, twisting and coiling like a snake, following the leader around the space.

3 Reverse this sequence of movements as near as possible, following the person at the other end of line as the leader.

4 Repeat with a new leader and a different method of travel, for example zig-zagging.

5 Ask for a volunteer, who then separates from the group.

6 The group continue but make their line into a knot, travelling around and under each other; when thoroughly knotted they freeze, but at no time unclasp hands.

7 The volunteer then attempts to untie the knot by physically maneouvring the group.

■Supplementary development of activity

1 Volunteer undoes knot by giving verbal instructions only to group.

2 Group undo own knot non-verbally.

■Additional outcome

Physical contact is engendered.

See page 236 for this activity used in another stage.

LEVEL 1

Aim: To promote range of movement between the three levels (*see Glossary*)

Population: Children

Conditions: None

Time: 5 minutes

Equipment: None

Structure: Individually, pairs

■Activity

1 Turn or spin at low level (ie on floor), for example on stomach, curled up on back, or sitting.
2 Turn or spin at medium level, eg. on knees.
3 Turn or spin at high level, eg. in a jump, on toes.
4 Leader to specify body parts taking the weight at first, then encouraging participants to find own.

■Supplementary development of activity

1 Find a partner and turn or spin together; assist each other to explore moving at each level, with different body parts taking the weight.
2 Make up a movement phrase together where each level is explored within turning or spinning movement.

■Additional outcomes

1 Adaptability within specific body activities of turning/spinning.
2 Awareness of the three levels of movement.

WARM-UP

VOCAL

Aim: To encourage sound and movement in combination

Population: Adults

Conditions: None

Time: 5–10 minutes (supplementary activity 20 – 30 minutes)

Equipment: None

Structure: Whole group

■Activity

1 Suggest participants inhale through their nose, take a deep breath and hum it out softly together.

2 Repeat with a louder hum until breath fully exhaled.

3 Repeat using sounds; 'ah, ooh, ee, la, ba, ra, ha, om'.

4 Use one of the sounds to initiate movement on the out breath.

■Supplementary development of activity

1 (a) Move from the sound 'la' and the base of the spine.
  (b) Move from the sound 'ba' and the centre of the body (below the navel).
  (c) Move from the sound 'ra' and the solar plexus (just above the navel).
  (d) Move from the sound 'ya' and the heart area of the body.
  (e) Move from the sound 'ha' and the throat area.
  (f) Move from the sound 'ah' and the middle of the brow area.
  (g) Move from the sound 'om' and the crown (top of the head).

2 Reverse the exercise above from (g) to (a).

3 Notice any images or colours that are associated with the sound/movement.

■Additional outcome

Control of breath and sound.

BREATH 1

Aim: To focus on the out breath
Population: All
Conditions: None — a prerequisite for vocal work
Time: 2–3 minutes
Equipment: None
Structure: Whole group

■Activity

1 Group stand in a circle — look towards the floor centre.
2 Leader suggests they close eyes and make a deep breath out.
3 Relax shoulders, arms and legs; bend slightly at the knees.
4 Allow breath to drift out slowly through the nose.
5 Repeat, allowing breath to drift out twice as slowly.

■Supplementary development of activity

1 Move arms on the out breath only, let the movement accompany the breath.
2 Move whole body on the out breath as a physical warm-up.

■Additional outcome

Concentration on breath helps to focus the participants, particularly with a view to inner movement and vocal work.

WARM-UP

BREATH 2

Aim: To enlarge vocalisation
Population: All
Conditions: Safety; not hurting
Time: 3 minutes
Equipment: None
Structure: Pairs

■Activity

1 Partner, with flat of hand, repeatedly makes short, quick slaps on the other's back.
2 Other expels sounds of 'mmm', 'ah', etc.
3 Reverse roles.

■Supplementary development of activity

Face partner and beat own chest with fists, expelling cries, opening mouth and throat so sound becomes louder.

BREATH 3

Aim: To encourage group to make sound
Population: All
Conditions: Some breath work in previous sessions
Time: 2 minutes
Equipment: None
Structure: Whole group

■**Activity**

1 Whole group relax at knees and take in deep breath.
2 Very slowly, let out breath and humming sound.
3 Allow sound to rise as eyes and arms lift to ceiling, until very loud.
4 Make movement shrink to floor; sound accompanies: sound and movement end simultaneously.

(Explain that some people may need more than one breath, and that they are able to breathe and make sound in own time.)

BREATH 4

Aim: To introduce sound and breath together
Population: All
Conditions: None
Time: 2 minutes
Equipment: None
Structure: Whole group

■Activity

1   Group can sit in circle.
2   All to breathe in through nose, make a huge yawn (no sound yet) and stretch arms.
3   Repeat with very slight sound.
4   Repeat noisily.
5   Divide group into three small groups; first group begins the yawn, second develops it, third finishes it, building up the sound per group.

■Supplementary development of activity

1   Repeat above, but with a sigh and any accompanying movement.
2   Make sigh longer and more noisy each time.

GENERAL SPACE

Aims: Imitation skills, getting to know the environment

Population: All

Conditions: First session

Time: 4–5 minutes

Equipment: Choice of music

Structure: Individual, pairs, small groups

■Activity

1   Individually the group move around the room, becoming familiar with the spaces, eg. corners, centre of the room, sides of the room.

2   Leader suggests they begin by walking slowly into and out of each space.

3   Next they jog through the space.

4   Finally they are encouraged to run into and out of the spaces.

5   Leader can suggest activities, for example jump when you feel you have left/arrived in a space, skip from/to each space, jog-walk, stop as you arrive to explore a space.

6   Ensure changes of speed and direction during activity.

7   In pairs. Partner A leads B through part of the previous journey, exploring the spaces in the room. Partner remains behind/beside and follows the movement activity exactly. Change leader.

8   Repeat the above in a small group, changing leader at leader's suggestion.

■Supplementary development of activity

1   Partners explore space as above with one leading and other following. Include gestures with hands as you go.

2   Change roles of leader and follower in own time without interrupting flow of movement.

3   Group leader moves and group follow.

■Additional outcomes

Turn-taking and experience of exploring space in room. Confidence in own movement and the space for moving through.

STRETCH 1

Aims: To identify and move body parts and muscle groups
Population: All
Conditions: Each session
Time: 5 minutes
Equipment: Music or percussion
Structure: Individual, partners

■Activity

1   Leader verbally identifies body parts in turn, and encourages a gradual stretch and release for each named part.
2   Change the levels for stretching, eg. lying, sitting, standing.
3   Use accompaniment if desired.

■Supplementary development of activity

Partner B stretches A's limbs gently while lying on floor.

■Additional outcomes

Awareness of sensation and articulation in body.

See page 239 for this activity used in another stage.

STRETCH 2

Aim: To warm body for later physical work

Population: All

Conditions: None

Time: 15 minutes

Equipment: Music

Structure: Pairs

■Activity

1 In pairs, stretch and relax a named body part in turn. Partner to echo.

2 Change energy level as progress is made through the body (ie begin very slowly). Leader could suggest they all move twice as slowly for the first 5–10 minutes.

■Additional outcome

Explore some new movements.

MASSAGE

Aims: To warm self and group; relaxation of muscles after physical exertion

Population: All

Conditions: None

Time: 5–10 minutes

Equipment: None

Structure: Whole group

■**Activity**

1 Make a close circle, sitting or standing; one behind gently massages the shoulders of one in front.

2 Turn around and repeat.

3 Each to give feedback on how soft/hard they want massage.

See page 238 for this activity used in another stage.

RELATIONSHIP 1

Aim: Initiating contact
Population: All
Conditions: None
Time: 2–5 minutes (depending on number in group)
Equipment: Bean bags or soft ball
Structure: Whole group

■Activity

1   Throw the bean bag gently to someone and say their name. They catch it and throw it to a different person, again saying their name, and so on.
2   Each person to have a turn at throwing. Can throw to same person more than once.
3   Repeat and say something about the person as bean bag is thrown.

■Additional outcome

Giving feedback.

RELATIONSHIP 2

Aims: To notice others' movements and imitate in own body

Population: All

Conditions: None

Time: Variable (1–4 minutes)

Equipment: None

Structure: Whole group

■Activity

1   In a circle one behind other, pass on the movement (given by leader). One behind copies the one in front. Let different movements emerge from the first one.

2   Repeat for 2–3 minutes, depending on the group's attention span.

PERSONAL SPACE 1

Aims: Impulse control and giving attention
Population: All
Conditions: None
Time: 4–5 minutes
Equipment: Music
Structure: Pairs

■Activity

1   Find and face a partner, sitting.
2   Decide who will be initiator and who the follower.
3   The initiator explores slowly the space immediately in front and between the twosome. They make shapes such as squares, circles and other pathways with their open hands through the air.
4   The partner follows, with their hands in a mirroring action.
5   At suggestion from leader they change roles several times while continuing to move.
6   Next the leader suggests they flow in and out of initiator and follower without stopping the movement, giving verbal hints as to when.
7   Repeat alone, giving non-verbal hints as to when.
8   Repeat without any hints.

■Supplementary development of activity

1   Change from sitting to kneeling and repeat above.
2   Change to standing or travelling and repeat.
3   Use other parts of the body, own choice or as suggested by leader, for initiating and mirroring movement.
4   Encourage physical contact between partners.

■Additional outcome

Turn-taking followed by a feeling sense of co-operation between partners as they learn to give and take as one.

RHYTHM 1

Aim: To create a structure for group
Population: All
Conditions: None
Time: 5–6 minutes
Equipment: None
Structure: Whole group

■Activity

1 Sitting in circle, leader claps out a simple rhythm and group copy.
2 Repeat with a more complex rhythm.
3 Volunteers take turns clapping out rhythm, group copy.

RHYTHM 2

Aim: To learn names
Population: All
Conditions: First meeting
Time: 5–10 minutes
Equipment: None
Structure: Whole group

■Activity

1 Sitting in a circle, leader claps out a simple rhythm eg. clap, clap, then says name.
2 Suggests whole group clap, clap and say names in interval between claps in turn around circle.
3 Repeat and reverse way round circle.

RHYTHM 3

Aim: To learn names
Population: All
Conditions: First session
Time: 5–10 minutes
Equipment: None
Structure: Whole group

■Activity

1 Sitting down in a circle, leader starts by saying own name, accompanied by claps for the number of syllables in the name.

2 Leader suggests whole group copies the clapping of each name three times as participants clap their own names out around the circle.

RHYTHM 4

Aim: To learn names
Population: All
Conditions: Early session
Time: 5 minutes
Equipment: None
Structure: Whole group

■Activity

1 Whole group sitting in a circle. Leader asks for suggestions for body sounds (non-vocal, such as clapping) from the group.

2 When 3 sounds have been suggested the leader puts them together to form a rhythm.

3 Group makes the rhythm and leader says their name in one of the intervals during it.

4 Whole group then continues with the rhythm, a name being said each time around the circle in turn at each repetition of the rhythm.

5 Repeat rhythm twice per person with group also saying name of each participant.

6 Repeat once per person — whole group says each name.

BODY CONTROL 3

Aim: To move whole body
Population: All
Conditions: None
Time: 5–10 minutes
Equipment: Music
Structure: Individual, partners

■Activity

1   Curl and stretch whole body.
2   Sway whole body.
3   Leap and jump with feet together and apart.
4   In partners, move with whole body activity to music. When music stops, one makes a shape, other copies.
5   Reverse roles.

BALANCE 3

Aim: To follow gross motor pattern of another, sustained movement quality

Population: All

Conditions: None

Time: 5–8 minutes

Equipment: Slow music

Structure: Pairs, small groups, large group

■Activity

1 Each person leads group in turn with a variety of balances.
2 Change balance on direction from group leader.
3 Repeat with a partner leading, changing balances in own time.
4 Followers to copy exactly the positions of stillness of partner.
5 Repeat as small then as large group, one balance then change leader.

■Supplementary development of activity

1 Same as above but travel between each balance in own pattern.
2 Balance as a pair/small group/large group after travelling (in physical contact).

■Additional outcomes

Containment of energy with others. Leadership and following skills. Creation of own movement forms and awareness of others. Working with music as an accompaniment.

BALANCE 4

Aims: To promote body/self control; to create own movement structure; to integrate something new into own structure

Population: All

Conditions: After well warmed-up

Time: 5–6 minutes

Equipment: Music if required (rhythmical)

Structure: Individual, pairs

■Activity

1 Hopping/jumping on the spot.
2 Change direction so as to travel forwards/backwards/sideways.
3 Make up own sequence of movement, exploring directions (eg. two in each direction.)

■Supplementary development of activity

1 After own sequence created, share with a partner, teach it.
2 Return to own space and use one or two of the movements just learned from partner and find place for them in your sequence.
3 Show partner finished sequence; partner to identify which part had been theirs.

■Additional outcomes

1 Can promote high energy in group.
2 Integration of a new movement into own pattern.
3 Awareness of how one movement can extend into different directions in space.
4 Sharing of movement.

BALANCE 1

Aims: To develop self-control and body awareness
Population: All
Conditions: None
Time: 4–5 minutes
Equipment: Music if desired
Structure: Individually and large group

■Activity

1   On spot in circle, move one isolated body part (for example, circling an arm). Leader begins by modelling movement.
2   After a few of these, give opportunity for participants to identify and articulate one body part in turn around the group. Say out loud the name of the body part and the type of articulation.

■Supplementary development of activity

1   Move two body parts.
2   Move one body part while rest of the body is in a specified shape, eg. kneeling, sitting, legs astride.

■Additional outcomes

1   Awareness in large group; turn-taking and following in rhythmic pattern.
2   Identification and articulation of body parts.

See page 74 for this activity used in another stage.

BALANCE 5

Aim: To reduce impulsivity

Population: All

Conditions: Adolescents may find blindfold more difficult

Time: 4–5 minutes

Equipment: Music, blindfold

Structure: Individually

■Activity

1 As in the game of 'statues', move with the music and freeze in a balance when it stops.

2 Leader identifies balance at first, eg. with one leg stretched behind.

3 Ask for a volunteer to 'stop' the music (with their back to the group).

4 Change volunteers.

5 After several turns, each member to create own balance.

6 On the 'stop', each member holds balance for 5 seconds, looks around and selects a balance from group for their next choice of balance.

■Supplementary development of activity

Repeat steps 1–4 blindfolded.

■Additional outcomes

1 Grounds (*see Glossary*) group and focuses them on centring (*see Glossary*) themselves.

2 Awareness of own and others' creativity.

3 Control of self and others (especially music operator).

See page 176 for this activity used in another stage.

BALANCE 6

Aims: Conforming to structure; assertion; fun

Population: All

Conditions: Reinforce ground rules of safety; no tickling or violence

Time: 20 seconds per shape; 10 minutes total

Equipment: None

Structure: Pairs

■Activity

1 In pairs, find own space, eg. on a mat.

2 Both warm up by walking on hands and feet in own space.

3 When feel comfortable in shape, freeze in it strongly.

4 Partner 'A' then attempts to unbalance their partner 'B' from their shape; partner 'A' can organise their energies in whatever way is best for unbalancing their partner.

5 Ensure both partners remain in specified shape for whole 20 seconds.

■Supplementary development of activity

1 Repeat 1–5 with another specified shape.

2 Repeat 1–5 while both squatting and jumping (remain in identified space).

■Additional outcomes

1 Contact via touch engendered.

2 Tolerance of frustration.

3 Awareness of own power stemming from body control and strength.

BALANCE 2

Aims: To develop control of body; to break 'rules'
Population: Children, adolescents, 'acting-out' adults
Conditions: Early sessions
Time: 5 minutes
Equipment: Drum
Structure: Individual

■Activity

1   Group at one side of room.
2   Walk across room and stop very still when hear drum, which beats rhythmically. Aim is to continue walking, beginning wherever they like, while drum still playing. Since the overt rule is to 'stay still until the drum stops', they must aim to break that rule. Leader to ensure they understand that the rule can be broken.
3   Hold stillness while drum continues.
4   Ask for volunteer to drum. They can make a guess at who will break the rule each time.

■Supplementary development of activity

1   Repeat, but run across room.
2   Repeat, but slide on belly across room.
3   Leader turns back on the group while drumming, so cannot see group.

■Additional outcome

Acknowledgement that 'rule-breaking' is possible in this structure.

See page 75 for this activity used in another stage.

LINES 1

Aim: To introduce concept of moving in space within a non-threatening structure

Population: All

Conditions: Early sessions

Time: 10 minutes

Equipment: Music — very slow, mystical

Structure: Individually

■Activity

1   Imagine a line drawing you out into space; draw it invisibly with your hand. Stretch out along it and back towards your centre.
2   Use all the directions, carve shapes in the air with this line.
3   Now use the surfaces of the body and other limbs to describe these shapes, exploring all the possibilities.

■Supplementary development of activity

1   In pairs, explore the qualities of your lines as one leads and the other follows (mirroring).
2   Perhaps give them some suggestions for lines, eg. short/long, curved/straight, continuous flow/interrupted flow, high/low.
3   Change leader.
4   Show the group some lines you have made on a large sheet of paper and have them all move whole body to each of these.

■Additional outcome

An awareness of their own and others' creativity.

RELATIONSHIP 3

Aims: To initiate, maintain and leave a relationship
Population: All
Conditions: None
Time: 3–5 minutes
Equipment: None
Structure: Pairs

■Activity

1   In pairs, one initiates slowly making contact with the other's hands to encourage swaying. Maintain contact, then say goodbye.
2   Change initiator; this time focus on a different body part, for example feet or shoulders.
3   After 2 above, both partners say goodbye and leave each other by moving away into a new space alone.

■Supplementary development of activity

1   Repeat 1–3 above and after leaving partner make contact with another person.
2   Repeat 1–3 with that person.

■Additional outcome

Receiving and gaining attention.

RELATIONSHIP 4

Aim: To assert an effect on the group

Population: All

Conditions: None

Time: 4–5 minutes

Equipment: Possibly music, if group lacking in confidence

Structure: Whole group

■Activity

1 In a circle, session leader leads the group in a 'do as I do' dance. Vary the speed, strength and body part.
2 In a line, repeat 1.
3 Travelling in a line, repeat 1.
4 Session leader could suggest changes in leadership or allow group to decide. Change leaders frequently (every 30–40 seconds).

QUALITY 1

Aim: To develop quality of strength
Population: All
Conditions: None
Time: 2–5 minutes
Equipment: Drum
Structure: Individual

■Activity

1   Leader suggests group imagine they are moving like a tiger stalking its prey.
2   On the sound of the drum they pounce on the prey.
3   Group gather strength to sound of drum then release it strongly in · pouncing movement.

QUALITY 2

Aim: To develop quality of strength

Population: Adolescents

Conditions: Safety ground rule

Time: 2–5 minutes

Equipment: Possibly tambourine

Structure: Individual

■Activity

Leader involves group in rehearsing 'Kung Fu'-like actions with arms and legs, encouraging jumping, kicking and turning.

■Supplementary development of activity

1   Remain on own mat.
2   Jump to the next mat with a 'Kung Fu' action.

QUALITY 3

Aim: To develop quality of lightness
Population: All
Conditions: None
Time: 2–5 minutes
Equipment: None
Structure: Individual

■Activity

1   Leader suggests group move as though a feather falling gently in the breeze.
2   Encourage circling, swaying, falling and floating movements in a quiet atmosphere.

■Supplementary development of activity

1   Only using hands and arms.
2   Only using feet and legs.

QUALITY 4

Aim: To introduce quality of suddenness
Population: All
Conditions: None
Time: 2–3 minutes
Equipment: None
Structure: Pairs

■Activity

1 Leader suggests labelling selves A and B.
2 Partner A then attempts to startle partner B by jumping, clapping and saying 'boo'. Partner ignores them.
3 Reverse roles.

■Additional outcome

Learning not to respond to provocation.

QUALITY 5

Aim: To introduce quality of suddenness
Population: Children, adolescents
Conditions: None
Time: 2 minutes
Equipment: Drum
Structure: Individual

■Activity

1 Leader suggests they move as though being shot by a machine-gun when drum sounds.
2 Encourage movement and stillness alternately.

QUALITY 6

Aim: To introduce sustained movement
Population: All
Conditions: None
Time: 2–3 minutes
Equipment: None
Structure: Pairs

■**Activity**

1 Leader suggests partner A moves arm in a gesture towards partner B.
2 Now make the same gesture at half the speed. Partner B watches intently as the gesture is made.
3 Now halve the speed again. Partner B gives feedback as to whether it seemed slower.
4 Finally, halve the speed again.
5 Reverse roles.

■**Additional outcome**

Focusing of attention.

BREATH 5

Aim: To energise and facilitate 'letting go'
Population: All
Conditions: Warmed up
Time: 1 minute
Equipment: None
Structure: Whole group

■Activity

1   Group in circle. Using elbows alternately, punch backwards, breathing out at same time.

2   Make a sound as breathe out.

PAIRS RESISTANCE 1

Aim: To introduce idea of going with as well as against another's resistance

Population: Adults, adolescents

Conditions: None

Time: 3–4 minutes

Equipment: None

Structure: Partners

■Activity

1 Find a partner; one stands behind the other, who is kneeling. Both face the front.
2 Make contact with hands.
3 Resist and go with partner's resistance alternately.
4 Ensure eyes are closed throughout activity.
5 The movement maintains an up-down direction as each partner flows in and out of their resistance.
6 Leader times the activity carefully, suggests change in roles.

■Supplementary development of activity

1 Facing partner, hand-to-hand contact, repeat 1–5 above.
2 Discussion with partner on theme of resisting, contact, etc.
3 Discussion with partner on what liked/disliked about interaction.

■Additional outcomes

1 Awareness of how participants individually contribute to or go with resistance from another.
2 How others affect our need to resist or flow with the direction of the resistance.

INTRODUCTION TO THEME

PAIRS RESISTANCE 2

Aim: To encourage personal strength

Population: All

Conditions: Repeat safety ground rules. First few sessions

Time: 10–15 minutes

Equipment: None

Structure: Pairs

■Activity

1 Partners sit back to back (backs in contact and knees bent) and, as leader counts aloud from 1 to 10, they push each other towards the other side of the room with all the strength they can muster.

2 Change partners, this time, standing and shoulder to shoulder (side to side).

3 Repeat pushing game with leader counting again and with other shoulders in contact.

4 Change partners again, this time hips to hips.

5 Change partners, hands to hands.

6 Change partners, hands to shoulders (making eye contact throughout).

■Supplementary development of activity

Could add a line between partners for them to attempt to push each other across.

■Additional outcomes

1 Should have 'resisted' almost every member of group by end of activity.

2 Having begun with the safer relationship (back to back) the group finish with a more open relationship (making eye contact and facing partner).

PERSONAL SPACE 2

Aim: Reaching through and receiving another in personal space

Population: Adults

Conditions: Some eye contact required, when group has become somewhat cohesive

Time: 4–5 minutes

Equipment: None

Structure: Large group

■Activity

1 Find a partner you feel you know and like. Number as 1 and 2.
2 1s make an outer circle around inner circle of 2s. Face partners and make eye contact.
3 Inner circle only, smile and reach with hands to receive contact with partner's hands.
4 Outer circle partners respond with smile and give hand contact.
5 Inner circle only, move round to the next person on right and repeat.
6 Continue to move round to right until returned to original partner.
7 Change inner and outer circles. Repeat with new people in the inner circle initiating contact.
8 Discussion in partners of any difficulties; what was the best thing about it, what did it remind you of?

■Supplementary development of activity

1 Repeat with a verbal greeting or name.
2 Repeat with eyes closed. Leader could ensure people unaware of who they were facing, that both reach out at the same time or give a choice, and give a longer time for hand contact with one or two participants only. Awareness could be stimulated by leader asking questions such as, 'can you tell if this person is male, female, outgoing, reticent?', etc.

■Additional outcomes

Members become more sensitive to each other and how they feel when people enter their personal space.

PERSONAL SPACE 3

Aim: To explore personal space
Population: Children, adults
Conditions: None
Time: 3 minutes
Equipment: Possibly music
Structure: Individual

■Activity

1 Leader suggests that participants imagine they are trapped in a net of some kind. Their task is to find a way out, but one part of their body (either given by the leader or their own choice) remains fixed to the floor throughout.

2 They are encouraged to imagine exploring the net to find a hole big enough to climb out through.

■Supplementary development of activity

1 Imagine another material enclosure on edge of personal space. Only by their reaching to furthest points around body does it become manifested.

2 Somewhere there is a gap in the enclosure through which to crawl. Leader could suggest the texture of the enclosure as being soft, glass, plastic, etc. Again emphasis is on the exploration around the body into the space immediately surrounding the participant, as far as they can reach while one part of the body is fixed to the wall/floor.

■Additional outcome

Heightened awareness of the movement opportunities within their own space.

PERSONAL SPACE 4
(Shadow Boxing)

Aim: To co-operate in a movement dialogue, taking turns
Population: Adolescents
Conditions: Reinforce safety rules
Time: 3 minutes
Equipment: None
Structure: Pairs, one behind and slightly to side of other

■Activity

1   Name of movement game is 'shadow boxing'; in pairs, A and B stand one behind the other.
2   A initiates a movement and freezes in a final shape, waits for B to imitate exactly.
3   A moves again, B imitates.
4   They turn to face the other way, this time B initiates.
5   Repeat for several turns.

■Supplementary development of activity

1   Make two or three movements each time but in slow motion.
2   Repeat exercise in a threesome.

■Additional outcomes

Some control of movement impulse and active management of waiting in turn-taking.

INTRODUCTION TO THEME

PERSONAL SPACE 5
(Space Action Dances)

Aims: To develop anticipation and prediction skills; awareness of the body in space

Population: Children and adolescents

Conditions: None

Time: 5–10 minutes

Equipment: None

Structure: Large group and pairs

■Activity

1   Name of activity is 'space action dances' (*see Laban movement analysis*). Start with large group sitting in a circle.

2   Leader moves arms, with an appropriate song, in the spatial planes, ie rocking side to side, up and down, forward and back, and all the way round.

3   Whole group sing and copy movements in rhythm.

4   Divide into pairs and move the dance together; change it in any way.

5   Share dance in fours when completed.

■Supplementary development of activity

1   Could involve more of body, eg. spin round on seat for 'all the way round'.

2   Practise sideways rolling in pairs or individually.

3   Forward/backward rolls individually on mats or from behind over partner or leader's back. The leader sits with legs astride catching roller as they bend over one shoulder and put hands on floor, curling in at waist, their head being protected as they are helped into and out of forward roll.

4   Spin around with partner, spin each other.

5   Jump with a partner, over a partner; in a threesome, two outsiders support and help the middle one from a low position to jump high off the ground and land back softly with knees bent.

6   Partners, when they have practised the above exercises, could choose three favourites and put them together so they flow one to the other.

■Additional outcomes

Awareness of spatial directions. Experience of body activities with the focus on which direction they move through.

SHAPES 1

Aims: To move and be still in group shaping

Population: Adolescents and adults

Conditions: None

Time: 5 minutes

Equipment: Could use music or percussion

Structure: Threes

■Activity

1 Label the three members A, B and C. A initiates by moving slowly and smoothly into a shape; B follows and fits with that shape, then C moves to fit with that shape. Hold shape for a few seconds.

2 Repeat the above with B leading, then C; thus members take turns to initiate, yet the group form a unified whole.

3 Discuss:
   (a) what you noticed
   (b) how you initiated
   (c) how you maintained the relationship.
   Is this a recognisable pattern?

■Supplementary development of activity

1 Repeat 1 and 2 above but this time with the As finding another group's A, meeting up and relating to them. The Bs and Cs stay attached, as though appendages, to their group's A, supporting the shape initiated.

2 Repeat 1 above but this time the two As find another two As from another group and relate to them. Bs and Cs stay supporting their own group's shape.

3 Repeat above until all As in the group are relating/interacting (non-verbally) with their supporters (Bs and Cs).

■Additional outcomes

1 An awareness of feeling unique, yet conforming to the group.

2 Acknowledgement of and support for the uniqueness of self.

3 An improvised choreography which the group maintains.

See page 160 for this activity used in another stage.

CHINESE WHISPERS

Aim: To practise imitation skills

Population: Adolescents, adults

Conditions: None

Time: 5 minutes

Equipment: None

Structure: Whole group or several small groups

■Activity

1   Group in circle standing one behind the other.

2   Leader gives instructions that each person should imitate any movement, however slight, that they notice the person in front making. No-one, however, is to move purposefully, other than to imitate the person in front.

3   The leader makes one purposeful movement to begin the group movement. The person behind the leader repeats it so that the movement is passed around the circle.

4   Allow group to experience the movements which evolve from all the unconscious movement emitted from members.

■Additional outcome

Awareness of how much movement we generate without full consciousness.

See page 185 for this activity used in another stage.

OBJECTS

Aims: To make an effect on the environment; to relate to an object; to work with anger

Population: All

Conditions: Early sessions, safety aspects reinforced

Time: 5–10 minutes

Equipment: Soft ball, football, netball, large table, chair

Structure: Individual, pairs

■Activity

1 After reinforcing safety aspects, give each member the opportunity to throw the ball against the wall.

2 Ensure an adequate distance away from the wall, give plenty of space between people. Begin with gentle throw developing into a strong, hard throw with all energy.

3 Regulate how they are to retrieve the ball.

4 What sound goes with the strong throw? All to make this at once.

5 What movement feels the most satisfying to make the throw?

6 In pairs, one to throw, the other to observe and retrieve ball. Encourage use of whole body, discuss in pairs what name might accompany the throw (someone from your life).

7 Share name in large group.

■Supplementary development of activity

1 Push or pull a large heavy object (eg. someone sitting on a chair, a table that is being pushed by others against the participant). Do this for a limited time period, eg. 20 seconds.

2 Discuss in pairs where/when this type of energy is used in each life and what happens next.

3 In turn, enact the scenario, beginning with the pushing and ending with own ending; use sound and words where they arise spontaneously.

4 Partner then moves the scenario in exactly the same way to show their partner a mirror of their movement story.

5 5 minutes to explore a different ending for self.

6 Enact new ending.

7 Discuss with partner how the exercise gave an understanding of patterns in our lives and to what extent learning about different use of self took place.

■Additional outcomes

Acknowledgement of anger. Recognition of a tension-provoking person in life and the patterns used to deal with frustration. Some insight into the effect they can make on others with their use of energy.

BRIDGES

Aim: To introduce contact

Population: All

Conditions: Not to be used if little body control

Time: 10–15 minutes

Equipment: None

Structure: Pairs, small groups

■Activity

1   One partner makes a bridge shape.
2   Partner moves under the bridge without touching it.
3   Any touch noticed by the bridge can result in them making a 'buzz' sound.
4   Change roles.
5   Repeat; this time touch is allowed.
6   Repeat with three different shapes.

■Supplementary development of activity

1   Partner to go over the bridge instead of under.
2   Groups of three or four make an 'over – under' shape together and volunteer moves through without/with touch. Repeat with new shape and new volunteer.   .

■Additional outcomes

Making physical contact without it predominating. Development of trust. Beginning to work on separation and merging with another.

IMAGERY

Aims: To engage with an image through movement; to stimulate the imagination; to encourage spontaneous movement

Population: All

Conditions: None

Time: 15–20 minutes

Equipment: Leader prepares drawn/written images on small pieces of paper

Structure: Individual, small groups

■Activity

1   Leader draws an image and shows it to the group, who then respond to it in movement for 20 seconds or so.

2   Leader folds up pieces of paper with drawn/written images upon them; each member selects one, then for 2 minutes explores the image in movement.

3   Repeat stage 2.

4   With a partner, try to guess the image from the movement responses.

5   Now each partner gives an image in turn for partner to respond to for 20 seconds. The image is given verbally, eg. 'move like a lion sneaking up on a deer'.

■Supplementary development of activity

1   In small groups, the leader secretly gives a visual or verbal image to each group.

2   Each group spends 4 minutes preparing to respond.

3   Each group shares their response with the whole group who may guess the image given.

■Additional outcomes

Development of symbolic expression, use of expressive movement in communication, development of a specific theme which the group is addressing, introduction of a relevant theme for the group.

See page 175 for this activity used in another stage.

BODY BOUNDARY 2

Aims: Centring, (*see Glossary*) self-assertion
Population: All
Conditions: None
Time: 15 minutes
Equipment: None
Structure: Partners

■Activity

1   Contract body inwards and hold tightly.
2   Partner tries to open up, but stay tightly closed. (Give a limited time for this, eg. 20 seconds, and state that there should be no violence or tickling.)
3   Change roles.
4   Offer a short discussion time on the issue of being closed off/someone wanting you to open up.

■Supplementary development of activity

1   Using fists only, partner this time attempts to open up the fist.
2   Both have eyes closed.

■Additional outcomes

1   Awareness of own strength and the development of a relationship with another group member.
2   Acknowledgement of need to remain closed at times.

BODY BOUNDARY 3

Aims: To give and receive peer attention; to develop trust, sensitivity and awareness of self affecting others

Population: Adolescents, adults

Conditions: Safety rules

Time: 10 minutes

Equipment: None

Structure: Pairs, whole group

■Activity

1   All stand in a circle.

2   Pummel all soft areas of own body and chest (making sound).

3   Pair up, one partner pummels with loose fists the other's calves, thighs, buttocks, backs, shoulders, upper arms.

4   Finish by stroking from the top of their head down to their feet slowly in one gentle sweep.

5   Repeat with a new partner (ie person on other side of you in the circle).

6   Notice the difference in contact between the two people who have massaged you. Notice your responses to them and any differences.

■Supplementary development of activity

1   After the above, open up a large group discussion which encourages each person to give feedback to those who massaged them.

2   Ask how it felt to be getting and giving this kind of attention from each other.

■Additional outcomes

A recognition of the part physical contact plays in their lives. A new level of relationship with peers. The ability to give and receive feedback from peers. Giving and receiving attention in a group.

See page 214 for this activity used in another stage.

BODY BOUNDARY 4

Aim: Differentiation of self from environment

Population: Adolescents, adults

Conditions: None

Time: 10 minutes

Equipment: None

Structure: Individual

■Activity

1   Lying on the floor. Move so that all the skin areas of your body come into contact with the floor.

2   Turn over and repeat.

3   Do not miss any areas, give them all a massage.

■Supplementary development of activity

1   Continue moving in contact with the floor but now with only your large muscles.

2   Move from one muscle group to another, exploring the balance as you go.

3   Now focus on the bones only.

4   Move so that joints and bones make contact with the floor; again balance as you go.

■Additional outcomes

Awareness of the periphery of the body through to the inner aspects of the body. Experience in stillness as balancing is worked with. Establishment of the floor as a friend and supporter.

BODY BOUNDARY 5

Aims: Differentiation of self from the environment, body awareness
Population: Adults
Conditions: None
Time: 10 minutes
Equipment: Gentle music
Structure: Individual

■Activity

1   Participants lie on the floor, keeping their eyes closed throughout the activity; they imagine they are floating in water, or through the air, their limbs gently supported.
2   Slowly move limbs, beginning with arms.
3   Carve a way through air or water and rise up to a standing position.
4   Begin to walk; carve shapes with limbs as travel through space.

■Supplementary development of activity

1   Imagine being in a different substance, such as glue, honey, or sand, carving shapes through it with arms, legs, body, head.
2   Repeat the activity with eyes open.
3   Use different sequences, for example, from standing to travelling to lying.

■Additional outcomes

1   Giving a sense of restrained flow.
2   Assertion of a clear air pattern through space.
3   Experiencing body boundaries and tension patterns.

FLOOR PATTERN 3

Aim: To say goodbye

Population: All

Conditions: End of session or period of treatment, or if a group member/leader is leaving

Time: 10–15 minutes

Equipment: Hoops or mats perhaps

Structure: Individual

■Activity

1 Make a straight, direct pathway toward one specific space in the room. Scan the room first and select somewhere.
2 Repeat, moving from space to space or object to object.
3 Repeat, moving from person to person.
4 Repeat all the above, but interacting non-verbally before leaving for next object/space/person.
5 Notice how long interaction takes and whether you initiate, maintain, respond or ignore interaction play. How do you leave?
6 Discuss in whole group:
   (a) how participants were left,
   (b) how they left others, spaces, objects.
   Notice any patterns/differences between people/objects/spaces. Relate to 'leaving' theme.

■Additional outcomes

Awareness of how leaving or being left can affect individuals and group.

INTRODUCTION TO THEME

LEVEL 3

Aims: To promote adaptability in movement and stillness between levels in space

Population: Children

Conditions: None

Time: 3 minutes

Equipment: Percussion if required

Structure: Individual

■Activity

1   Make a high shape and hold it before spiralling down to the floor, sinking slowly into it as you arrive.

2   Explore spirals from high to low and low to high.

3   Make stops at three different places on the spiral.

4   Make two stops on the way up the spiral and three stops on the way down. Choice of how long these stops take.

■Supplementary development of activity

1   Vary the speed of the spiral so as to experience stillness from sustained and sudden movement.

2   Ensure same/different shape in stillness each time.

3   Repeat all the above with a partner or in a threesome, complementing stillnesses.

4   Leader could direct the whole activity so that all participants are moving and stopping at one time.

■Additional outcomes

Some decision-making skills used in choice of when and for how long to stop in stillness. Body control and extension of movement range.

LEVEL 3

Aims: To engender co-operation in small group; to encourage movement/experience in the high level

Population: Adolescents/adults

Conditions: Warmed up physically

Time: 2–3 minutes

Equipment: None

Structure: Threes

■Activity

1   Groups of three, volunteer stands in middle, other two either side supporting the middle one under arms and at forearms/hands.

2   Two outsiders assist middle one to jump up; they begin and land with knees bent.

3   Repeat with new person in the middle.

■Additional outcomes

1   Support of another.

2   Experience jumping with assistance.

3   Energising for whole group.

AIR PATTERN 1

Aim: To use an object as an extension of the self

Population: All

Conditions: None

Time: 4–5 minutes

Equipment: Pieces of fabric, of various shapes, colours, sizes and weights

Structure: Individual

■Activity

1   Each participant selects a piece of fabric.
2   Explore its properties by moving it in space, on the spot and travelling.
3   Use it to carve out shapes in the air while on the spot.
4   Use it to carve out shapes in the air while travelling and changing directions in space.

■Supplementary development of activity

1   Move on the floor with the fabric.
2   Use it as a magic carpet and take a journey with it for 2 minutes.
3   Move with a partner and with fabric.
4   Using one very large piece of fabric work in fours or the whole group, with focus on moving with fabric.

BODY SHAPE

Aim: To develop awareness of the body shape in space

Population: Children

Conditions: None

Time: 4–5 minutes

Equipment: Possibly music/percussion

Structure: Individual, partners

■Activity

1   Leader gives direction for all participants to make their bodies
into a specific shape, for example:
    (a) like a ball — as *round* as you can,
    (b) like a wall — as *wide* as you can,
    (c) like a lamppost — as *tall* as you can,
    (d) like a giant — as *big* as you can,
    (e) like a ladybird — as *small* as you can,
    (f) like a twig — as *crooked* as you can.

■Supplementary development of activity

1   Repeat (a)–(f) above in pairs. Encourage physical contact.
2   Give shapes to each pair, eg. star, cross, spiral, letters.
3   Repeat step 2 above but in threes or fours, and ask them to spell
out a simple name from the group (eg. John).
4   Small group could move into any shape above, from eg. walking,
running, jumping, skipping, using music/percussion for travelling
steps, then leader stopping it for groups to make shapes. Groups
could see who got into specified shape first.

■Additional outcomes

Emphasis on shapes such as pointed, angular, round, twisted, as an
individual, in twos, and within a group.

DIRECTIONALITY 1

Aims: Movement imitation, turn-taking, giving of attention

Population: All

Conditions: None

Time: 5 minutes

Equipment: Music if desired

Structure: Small groups (4–5)

■Activity

1   All standing in a line, one behind the other.
2   Leader of line moves one arm sideways and those behind copy at the same time.
3   Leader moves both arms and all copy.
4   Leader moves legs and/or arms for all to copy.
5   Change leader.

■Supplementary development of activity

1   Leader travels, using only feet.
2   Whole group become one line (the small groups join up).

PIN ROLL

Aim: To be effective with others

Population: All

Conditions: Give enough space to each pair

Time: 10 minutes

Equipment: None (could make a 'goal' at one end for partner to roll towards)

Structure: Pairs

■**Activity**

In pairs, roll partner along floor in a pin roll (arms stretched out above head). Use different body parts, such as feet, head, hands, to propel partner.

■**Supplementary development of activity**

1 Could roll individually in pin rolls across the floor.
2 Hold hands with a partner and roll together.

BODY CONTROL 4

Aims: To be aware of movement and stillness

Population: All

Conditions: None

Time: 4–5 minutes

Equipment: Light classical music, if desired

Structure: Individual

■Activity

1   Rhythm of walking and being still suggested; eg. walk, walk, still, still.

2   Each participant makes own rhythm of being still and walking.

■Additional outcome

Development of internal control.

PRE-LATERALITY 1

Aim: Co-ordinate arms and legs in rhythm
Population: All
Conditions: None
Time: 5–8 minutes
Equipment: Marching music if desired, drums
Structure: Individually, whole group

■Activity

1 Marching with same arms and legs, ie both right arm and leg move together then both left arm and leg.
2 Marching with opposite arms to legs (ie right arm with left leg — it may be better, though, not to mention right and left specifically).
3 March in whole group with different leaders.
4 Could incorporate drummers accompanying marchers.
5 Leader could clap out rhythm.

■Supplementary development of activity

1 Create own phrase individually using arm/leg co-ordination and march it out around the room.
2 Half group share with other half and change over.

■Additional outcome

Development of awareness of the two sides of the body.

145

PRE-LATERALITY 2

Aim: Body awareness
Population: All
Conditions: None
Time: 5–6 minutes
Equipment: Ribbon, material
Structure: Individually, partners

■Activity

1 Lying on back, move in co-ordination arms and legs, opening and closing; leader directs.
2 The partner who is lying watches the partner who is standing up in front of them and copies movement of arms and legs as though a mirror.
3 Leader may suggest shaking of one hand, kicking one leg, as well as two arms and/or two legs moving together.
4 Partner is only to use one side of body now — identify by tying material, ribbon, or giving to hold.
5 Change roles.

■Supplementary development of activity

1 Repeat 1–5 with both standing up facing each other.
2 Repeat 1–5 with one behind the other.
3 Repeat 1–5 with partners side by side.

■Additional outcomes

Stress of one side of the body and then the other.

See page 170 for this activity used in another stage.

FALLING

Aim: To develop sense of 'giving in' to gravity

Population: Adolescents, adults

Conditions: After some trust between participants established

Time: 4–5 minutes

Equipment: None

Structure: Whole group, partners

■Activity

1   In a line, one in front of the other, close together. The second participant down the line (the catcher) places their arms around the first participant from behind.

2   The first participant then gently and slowly allows their ankles, knees and hips to collapse and they fall against their catcher. Catcher ensures they fall against them and slide down them to the floor.

3   The catcher takes as much weight from the faller as appropriate. Faller lets go into the floor.

4   The third participant (the next catcher) then moves forward and places themselves close to the body of the next faller (the previous catcher).

5   Repeat falling and catching until all in the line have fallen to the floor, and then the last one in the line turns around; the others stand up; and the whole activity is repeated, starting from the back of the line.

■Supplementary development of activity

1   Partners can practise the roles of catcher and faller.

2   Discussion about being caught, letting go, falling and catching.

■Additional outcomes

1   A 'letting go' of the physical and emotional self.

2   Trusting self enough to be safe in the arms of another.

3   Trusting self to catch, hold and take care of another.

AIR PATTERN 2

Aims: To identify self and make own shapes in air pattern
Population: Children
Conditions: None
Time: 2 minutes
Equipment: None
Structure: Individually

■Activity

1 Each participant sitting down draws out letter shapes in the air as suggested by the leader.
2 Make the letter shapes bigger, use a larger area of space so you have to move.
3 Repeat, drawing out own name.
4 Repeat, drawing out another group member's name.
5 Repeat, drawing out one word.

■Supplementary development of activity

Partner could guess the word/name.

AIR PATTERN 3

Aim: To encourage movement of limbs in space

Population: All

Conditions: None

Time: 4 minutes

Equipment: Possibly abstract music

Structure: Individual

■Activity

1 All participants move in space, carving out shapes in the air with arms, then legs, then head only.

2 Repeat, co-ordinating limbs and other surfaces of body as you carve way through space.

■Additional outcomes

1 Assert own movement in space.

2 Make an effect on the environment.

MASKS

Aim: To promote awareness of masks in life

Population: Adults/adolescents

Conditions: Once safety and trust are established in the group

Time: 40 minutes – 1 hour

Equipment: A variety of objects

Structure: Individual

■Activity

1 Bring to the session a variety of objects provided by participants and/or leader.

2 Each participant makes a mask to go over face and/or head. Spend about 30 mins on this.

3 Using the mask, explore sitting/kneeling/standing positions for this mask. If large mirrors are available have group face mirror for these explorations.

4 Next have group move in steps to a repetitive rhythm which is representative of the mask. If using mirrors have them face front all the time and move across space in front of mirror in turn.

5 Partners. Share an improvisation in turn where you use the positions and step pattern. Partner to watch and be aware of how it makes you feel.

6 Discuss what you felt as you observed your partner. What masks did you use? What are you hiding behind these?

■Supplementary development of activity

Imagine drinking a potion which affects the body. Explore in mask how the potion makes participants move, eg. cold, numb, heavy, rigid, frozen as though a stone.

■Additional outcome

An awareness of how masks can hide/reveal the inner self.

BREATH 6

Aims: To focus on in and out breath in movement
Population: Adults
Conditions: None
Time: 5–10 minutes
Equipment: Meditation or healing music
Structure: Whole group

■Activity

1   Leader suggests group sit/lie in own space, eyes closed.
2   Focus on out breath, breathing out through nose and relaxing body several times, use evenly the whole of the chest and abdomen to expel air slowly.
3   Focus on in breath (through nose); slowly allow air to enter abdomen and chest region.
4   Focus on pause between in and out or out and in breaths. Be aware of what part of your breath cycle has the pause/still point.
5   Begin to move as an accompaniment to:
(a) out breath,
(b) in breath,
(c) pause.
Aim to rise to standing and travelling in own time.

■Supplementary development of activity

Breathe out as though through toes and other areas of the body, eg. backs. Imagine every cell of the body expanding as you exhale through the nose.

■Additional outcomes

Inner focus encouraged, awareness of body in co-ordination and movement as an accompaniment of the breath.

INTRODUCTION TO THEME

TRUST 1

Aim: To develop trust in group
Population: All
Conditions: Early in sessions, safety rules emphasised
Time: 10–15 minutes
Equipment: None
Structure: Partners

■Activity

1 Partners catch each other in turn but only when the 'faller' decides to fall against catcher.
2 Catcher is to ensure feet are on wide base, one behind the other and knees bent slightly; hands wide, ready to catch partner by shoulder blades as they fall backwards.
3 Faller to stand 6 to 10 inches away at first, then gradually extend distance of fall. Keep body rigid. Catcher simply catches and returns them to upright position.
4 Reverse roles.

■Supplementary development of activity

Repeat above with faller falling towards partner, partner catches them by the front of their shoulders.

■Additional outcome

Trusting own weight to another.

INTRODUCTION TO THEME

BODY CONTROL 5

Aims: To promote awareness, rhythm and impulse control

Population: All

Conditions: None

Time: 3 minutes

Equipment: Strong, rhythmic music

Structure: Whole group

■**Activity**

1   Group sit on floor and rock backwards and forwards, hands behind head.
2   The music is then played and group rock in time.
3   At several points leader stops music, when the group have to freeze in their positions.
4   Leader needs to vary the length of the pauses between playing the music.

INTRODUCTION TO THEME

RHYTHM 5

Aim: Imitation skills

Population: All

Conditions: None

Time: 5 minutes

Equipment: None

Structure: Partners

■**Activity**

1   In partners, one gently taps out a simple rhythm on the back of the other, who then stamps/claps back the same rhythm.
2   Reverse roles.
3   Repeat with more complex rhythms.

INTRODUCTION TO THEME

RHYTHM 6

Aim: Awareness of inner rhythm
Population: All
Conditions: None
Time: 5 minutes
Equipment: A drum each
Structure: Whole group

■Activity

1 Participants to engage in vigorous activity, then place hand on pulse/heart to feel the beat.
2 Drum out the rhythm.
3 Stamp out the rhythm.
4 Clap out the rhythm.

SHAPES & WORDS

Aims: To explore emotions and associated postures in a group

Population: All

Conditions: None

Time: 5 minutes

Equipment: None

Structure: Threes

■Activity

1   Leader says 3 words in turn that describe emotions (eg. joy, fear, etc).

2   For each word in turn, each group member takes a turn to make a shape in the centre of the circle. The other two members complement it, so that the whole group shape represents the emotion.

3   Leader indicates when each member is to take up the shape by saying '1,2,3' for each word.

ROCK

Aim: To hold own ground
Population: All
Conditions: No violence
Time: 2 minutes
Equipment: None
Structure: Pairs

■Activity

1   For one member of each pair, leader says 'make yourself like a rock'. Encourage use of wide base, low to the floor.
2   Partner attempts to push them over.
3   Change over.

■Supplementary development of activity

Do with several partners.

■Additional outcomes

1   Self-assertion.
2   Development of the quality of strength with bound flow (*see Laban movement analysis*).

LOCOMOTION 1

Aims: To move in accordance with a set rhythm, travelling (*see Glossary*) in a co-ordinated, rhythmic experience

Population: Children, adults

Conditions: None

Time: 10 minutes

Equipment: Drum, music of your choice

Structure: Whole group as individuals, in partners, trios

■Activity

1   Leader beats out a rhythm on the drum or puts on the music.
2   Leader varies the rhythm and calls out ways of travelling (eg. walk, gallop, slide, jump, slither).

■Supplementary development of activity

1   Join up with a partner and follow the pattern of travelling the partner selects, while leader continues to beat out a rhythm; then repeat, reversing roles.
2   Repeat in trios, small groups, periodically changing the person deciding the pattern.
3   Let a volunteer beat out rhythm on drum or select the music for the group.

■Additional outcomes

1   More trust develops as the leader is accepted.
2   All members can initiate their own ideas for travelling within the safety of a clear rhythmic pattern.
3   The group learns to follow the lead from others and turn taking is experienced in taking the lead.

See page 76 for this activity used in another stage.

LOCOMOTION 4

Aim: To encourage forms of locomotion

Population: All

Conditions: None

Time: 5–10 minutes

Equipment: None

Structure: Whole group

■Activity

1   Leader suggests group walk around space in readiness for a movement activity suggested by a volunteer.

2   At any point in time a participant (selected by leader or self-selected) can call out a travelling activity (eg. hop, jump, roll, etc).

3   The group continue the specified activity until another volunteer participant calls out an activity, at which point the group moves in that manner.

4   Repeat so that all members have been 'caller volunteers', whether spontaneously or at direction of leader.
(There is no need for 'callers' to drop out of the group's movement.)

■Additional outcome

Participants have opportunity to lead group.

SHAPES 2

Aims: To explore characteristics and/or emotions associated with postures in a group

Population: All

Conditions: None

Time: 10–15 minutes

Equipment: None

Structures: Threes or fours

■Activity

1 In turn each member (the initiator) takes up a shape in the centre which expresses how they feel, or one unique characteristic of themselves.

2 Rest of the group silently ask themselves 'What is being expressed? Does this person need physical support? Distance? Touch?'

3 Then each group member chooses to enter that space or not. Once they have entered they respond to the person's shape with another; they may add to it as seems appropriate, then leave.

4 The initiator returns to the group when they feel there have been enough responses.

5 Group ask what was especially satisfying. Initiator asks group what they thought he was communicating to them. Initiator tells group how he felt they responded. Group ask themselves what their role was (eg. support, self-interest, etc).

■Supplementary development of activity

Repeat in whole group, using centre of circle for each to enter in turn.

■Additional outcomes

1 To be part of a group yet separate from it.

2 Expression of 'differentness' and that being accepted.

SHAPES 1

Aims: To move and be still in group shaping

Population: Adolescents and adults

Conditions: None

Time: 5 minutes

Equipment: Could use music or percussion

Structure: Threes

■Activity

1   Label the three members A, B and C. A initiates by moving slowly and smoothly into a shape; B follows and fits with that shape, then C moves to fit with that shape. Hold shape for a few seconds.

2   Repeat the above with B leading, then C; thus members take turns to initiate, yet the group form a unified whole.

3   Discuss:
   (a) what you noticed
   (b) how you initiated
   (c) how you maintained the relationship.
   Is this a recognisable pattern?

■Supplementary development of activity

1   Repeat 1 and 2 above but this time with the As finding another group's A, meeting up and relating to them. The Bs and Cs stay attached, as though appendages, to their group's A, supporting the shape initiated.

2   Repeat 1 above but this time the two As find another two As from another group and relate to them. Bs and Cs stay supporting their own group's shape.

3   Repeat above until all As in the group are relating/interacting (non-verbally) with their supporters (Bs and Cs).

■Additional outcomes

1   An awareness of feeling unique yet conforming to the group.

2   Acknowledgement of and support for the uniqueness of self.

3   An improvised choreography which the group maintains.

See page 127 for this activity used in another stage.

SHAPES 3

Aims: To move within a group, initiating and maintaining a relationship with each other.

Population: Adults

Conditions: None

Time: 8–10 minutes

Equipment: Music

Structure: Two groups

■Activity

1   Divide into two groups and label selves A, B, C etc.

2   To the accompaniment of music, A goes into the centre of the group and makes a shape (*see Laban Movement Analysis*); then, by stretching, reaching and twisting, they move into a second shape.

3   As they make their transition from the first shape to the second, person B joins in and moves to make a linked shape with A's second shape.

4   Then A and B move together slowly to make a third shape, while person C joins in.

5   Keep moving and incorporate each group member until a mobile sculpture evolves, where all the group are moving and connecting, filling spaces and levels.

6   Bring it to a close at the end of the music by asking the group to find a final shape and freeze.

SHAPES 4

Aims: To introduce emotions and their associated postures

Population: All

Conditions: None

Time: 5 minutes

Equipment: None

Structure: Twos, threes

■**Activity**

1 Ask each group to suggest an emotion to you. Label group members 1 and 2 (and 3 if in threes).

2 Explain that you will call out one of these emotions in turn and each no. 1 will respond with a reflection of the emotions in a posture.

3 Each no. 2 supports the posture with their own posture, followed by no. 3.

4 Change numbers in the group and repeat with next emotion, etc.

TRUST 2

Aim: To develop trust
Population: All
Conditions: Safety ground rule
Time: 5–10 minutes
Equipment: None
Structure: Threes

■Activity

1   Catch a middle person who decides when they will fall between the two others standing either side.
2   Ensure the catchers stand safely to receive the weight. One will catch the faller from behind, one from in front.
3   Change roles and each have turn as different catcher and as faller.
4   Extend space gradually between faller and catchers.

■Supplementary development of activity

1   Repeat above, but with faller's eyes closed.
2   Repeat above, but with faller passive. Catchers catch and push back to other catcher rather than to middle balance position.

■Additional outcomes

Excitement at risk taking. Confidence at ability to support others.

DEVELOPMENT OF THEME

TRUST 3

Aim: To develop ability to 'let go' of others and 'catch' self and others

Population: All

Conditions: Safety rule

Time: 15–25 minutes

Equipment: None

Structure: Threes

■Activity

1 No.1 (faller) faces no.2 (holder) and takes wrist contact with opposite hand, holding no.2 and leaning back so that weight is taken by contact. No.3 (catcher) takes up position close behind no.1.

2 Faller then counts '1,2,3' then lets go of wrist of no.2 and is caught by no.3.

3 Reverse roles so all take turn in each of the three roles.

4 In threes, discuss each role — how was it to be in each, for each person?

■Supplementary development of activity

1 Repeat above, but with no.2 counting '1,2,3' and letting go of faller. Holder takes opposite wrist of faller who does not hold on. Repeat with faller's eyes closed. Repeat without catcher (faller has to catch self).

2 Repeat 1–3, but with faller's eyes closed. Repeat without catcher.

■Additional outcomes

1 Development of free flow to bound flow (*see Laban movement analysis*).

2 Taking risks and containing self.

TRUST 4

Aim: . To engender group trust
Population: All
Conditions: Safety rules, early in sessions
Time: 10–15 minutes
Equipment: None
Structure: Whole group

■**Activity**

1 Group stand in circle, close together, shoulder to shoulder, hands flat and at shoulder height, one foot in front of other.
2 Volunteer (faller) stands rigid in centre and falls towards others who catch them gently and slowly by their shoulder blades and move them across to next person in circle.
3 Change volunteer.

■**Supplementary development of activity**

1 Repeat, volunteer with eyes closed.
2 Repeat with more distance between catchers and fallers.
3 Could begin by requesting that volunteer decides when to fall and where. Catchers simply place them back in centre after each fall.
4 Repeat with fallers deciding to sink into floor, roll and get up, before falling against others again. Catchers support all movements.

■**Additional outcomes**

1 Physical contact for whole group.
2 'Letting go' in the group.
3 Being moved by others.
4 Self-trust.

RHYTHM 7

Aim: To create a rhythmical movement phrase

Population: All

Conditions: None

Time: 5–10 minutes

Equipment: None

Structure: Whole group

■**Activity**

1 Leader or group member suggests several words or phrases in turn.

2 Participants as a group chant and clap them out.

3 Participants select one of the words or phrases to individually move to in rhythm. Break it down into syllables.

4 In partners, share the moving rhythm — partner tries to guess which word/phrase it is based on.

LEVEL 4

Aims: To promote wider vocabulary of movement and adaptation of movements to different levels (*see Glossary*)

Population: Children

Conditions: None

Time: 2–3 minutes

Equipment: None

Structure: Individually

■Activity

1 Leader suggests the upper part of the body is opened and stretched at a specific level (*see Glossary*); for example, stretching out arms horizontally while standing would be a stretch at the medium level.

2 Repeat this opening movement with the upper body, but at another level; for example, the same stretch as above while lying down.

3 Now close and curl the upper part of the body at a specified level.

4 Repeat this closing movement at another level.

■Supplementary development of activity

1 Close upper and open lower part of the body, each at different levels, for example twist and hug the upper body while standing with feet wide apart.

2 Open upper and close lower part of the body, each at different levels.

■Additional outcome

Co-ordination between upper and lower parts of the body.

See page 229 for this activity used in another stage.

LEVEL 5

Aim: To promote adaptability in movement
Population: All
Conditions: Mats underneath groups, safety element emphasised
Time: 5–10 minutes
Equipment: Mats
Structure: Groups of 4–8

■Activity

1   Leader suggests group size, depending on age/functioning.
2   A volunteer lies down on back and the group carefully kneel each side, hands joining in criss-cross pattern, wrist to wrist under shoulders, hips and legs of volunteer.
3   Leader ensures firm support (including the head and arms) before group lift volunteer to a high level, above the supporters' heads if possible.
4   They keep the support and hold the volunteer at a low level before carefully placing him on the ground.

■Supplementary development of activity

1   A swaying movement at both levels may be made by group if safe support is still possible.
2   Whole group help to lift and lower a volunteer.

■Additional outcomes

1   Volunteer experiences their supported body at two levels.
2   Group experience their ability to work together to support the full body weight of the member.

LEVEL 6

Aim: To promote development of internal structure
Population: Children
Conditions: Warmed up physically
Time: 2–3 minutes
Equipment: Lively music
Structure: Individually

■Activity

1   Leader suggests a practice activity, jumping, then jumping and turning in the air. Teach 'giving in to the floor' on landing from jumps.
2   Exploration of jumping and turning at high, medium and low levels follows.
3   Each participant makes a short 'jumping and turning' dance; ie they select three or four movements they like to make and put them together, flowing from one to the next.

■Supplementary development of activity

1   Share the finished dance in threes.
2   Find a way for the three dances to be joined together so that they are integrated.

■Additional outcomes

1   Creation of own structure for a particular movement activity at different levels.
2   Some energising of the group as a whole.

PRE-LATERALITY 2

Aim: Body awareness
Population: All
Conditions: None
Time: 5–6 minutes
Equipment: Ribbon, material
Structure: Individually, partners

■Activity

1 Lying on back, move in co-ordination arms and legs, opening and closing; leader directs.
2 The partner who is lying watches the partner who is standing up in front of them and copies movement of arms and legs as though a mirror.
3 Leader may suggest shaking of one hand, kicking one leg as well as two arms and/or two legs moving together.
4 Partner is only to use one side of body now — identify by tying material, ribbon, or giving to hold.
5 Change roles.

■Supplementary development of activity

1 Repeat 1–5 with both standing up facing each other.
2 Repeat 1–5 with one behind the other.
3 Repeat 1–5 with partners side by side.

■Additional outcomes

Stress of one side of the body and then the other.

See page 146 for this activity used in another stage.

PRE-LATERALITY 3

Aim: To restrict movement to one side of the body, not crossing mid-line

Population: Children

Conditions: None

Time: 3 minutes

Equipment: Marker pens

Structure: Individually, partners

■Activity

1 Leader tells group, 'imagine you had an opportunity to drive a car'.

2 The group then mime, with leader direction, getting into the car and starting it up.

3 Tell the group members that they are not allowed to turn the wheel so far round that their arms cross over their body mid-line; identify this by shirt buttons, etc.

4 Give them directions as though map reading to a blind driver, eg. 'turn left slowly (big bend), straight on down the hill, turn sharp right, over traffic lights, stop, straight on, round the roundabout to the right, then come off to the left'.

5 Perhaps give mark on a hand to help them distinguish right from left.

6 The group travel physically during mime.

■Supplementary development of activity

Repeat 1–6 with partner in passenger seat giving map reading directions.

■Additional outcomes

Identification of right from left in body and in movement.

BODY CONTROL 6

Aim: To develop response to others' needs
Population: All
Conditions: Well into session
Time: 10–15 minutes
Equipment: None
Structure: Individual, partners

■Activity

1   Individually group members balance on parts of the body, changing point of contact with floor after each balance; movement flows on.
2   Partners (A and B). Partner A finds ways of assisting partner B in balances they choose. Leader teaches support of partner for safety.
3   Partners counterbalance each other so that they can sit down, wrists in contact with each other.
4   Explore in trios counterbalance ideas.

■Additional outcomes

Sensitivity to own body weight and its supportive aspects.

FLOOR PATTERN 4

Aims: To develop spatial orientation, decision making, turn-taking, trust

Population: Children

Conditions: None

Time: 4 minutes

Equipment: None

Structure: Whole group

■Activity

1 Group take up individual shapes.
2 Two volunteers act as travellers, one leading, one following, and move over, around and under others in twisting pathways, staying close together.
3 Group leader suggests a variety of speeds and methods of travel.
4 The one leading can decide to give follower the lead by taking on any other group member's shape. That group member then becomes the follower.

■Supplementary development of activity

1 Have three or four volunteers as the travellers.
2 Perhaps add music to accompany the dancing journey.

■Additional outcome

Tolerance of frustration for those not immediately chosen to become followers.

FLOOR PATTERN 5

Aims: To arrive/leave with a flexible pathway
Population: All
Conditions: Beginning of group series/end of group series
Time: 10–15 minutes
Equipment: None
Structure: Individuals, partners

■Activity

1 Each participant takes a circular, meandering pathway towards a space/object/person. Repeat for 3 minutes, travelling through several paths.

2 Select three pathways to approach and leave spaces/objects/ people. Travel in variety of ways across floor.

3 Rehearse each pathway and put them together to make a dance which focuses on arrival at and leaving the selected spaces/ objects/people.

4 Share in twos the final pathway.

5 Discuss in twos what was noticed about partner's approach and arrival, then departure from selected places.

■Supplementary development of activity

1 Whole group discussion about flexibility of approach and departure and what that conjures up for participants about their expectations for the group.

2 Explore direct pathways to/from places.

■Additional outcomes

1 Arrival/departure issues acknowledged.

2 Contrasting pathways explored.

IMAGERY

Aims: To engage with an image through movement; to stimulate the imagination; to encourage spontaneous movement

Population: All

Conditions: None

Time: 15–20 minutes

Equipment: None

Structure: Individual, small groups

■Activity

1 Leader draws an image and shows it to the group, who then respond to it in movement for 20 seconds or so.

2 Leader folds up pieces of paper with drawn/written images upon them; each member selects one, then for 2 minutes explores the image in movement.

3 Repeat stage 2.

4 With a partner, try to guess the image from the movement responses.

5 Now each partner gives an image in turn for partner to respond to for 20 seconds. The image is given verbally, eg. 'move like a lion sneaking up on a deer'.

■Supplementary development of activity

1 In small groups, the leader secretly gives a visual or verbal image to each group.

2 Each group spends 4 minutes preparing to respond.

3 Each group shares their response with the whole group who may guess the image given.

■Additional outcomes

Development of symbolic expression, use of expressive movement in communication, development of a specific theme which the group is addressing, introduction of a relevant theme for the group.

See page 132 for this activity used in another stage.

BALANCE 5

Aim: To reduce impulsivity
Population: All
Conditions: Adolescents may find blindfold more difficult
Time: 4–5 minutes
Equipment: Music, blindfold
Structure: Individually

■Activity

1 As in the game of 'statues', move with the music and freeze in a balance when it stops.
2 Leader identifies balance at first, eg. with one leg stretched behind.
3 Ask for a volunteer to 'stop' the music (with their back to the group).
4 Change volunteers.
5 After several turns, each member to create own balance.
6 On the 'stop', each member holds balance for 5 seconds, looks around and selects a balance from group for their next choice of balance.

■Supplementary development of activity

Repeat steps 1–4 blindfolded.

■Additional outcomes

1 Grounds group and focuses them on centring themselves (*see Glossary*).
2 Awareness of own and others' creativity.
3 Control of self and others (especially music operator).

See page 108 for this activity used in another stage.

TENSION–RELAXATION 1

Aim: To use imagination in association with tension-release activity

Population: Children, adolescents

Conditions: None

Time: 3 minutes

Equipment: None

Structure: Individual

■Activity

1   Move like 'Action Man' with strong, jerky actions.
2   Transform into 'floppy doll' with flaccid movements.
3   Have group go from one interpretation to the other rapidly in turn (eg. 10 seconds in each alternately).

■Additional outcome

Adaptation in movement.

TENSION–RELAXATION 2

Aims: To promote body sensation and self-trust
Population: All
Conditions: Warmed up
Time: 3–4 minutes
Equipment: None
Structure: Individual

■**Activity**

1   Sitting with one leg bent under hips, gently support self as you lie back slowly.
2   Feel muscles in thigh stretching, breathe out as though into them and relax back on elbows.
3   If able, go further back for 30 seconds and watch breath.
4   Slowly come back up to sitting and repeat on other side.

QUALITY 7

Aim: To develop quality of strength
Population: All
Conditions: None
Time: 2–5 minutes
Equipment: None
Structure: Individual, group

■Activity

1 Leader suggests a mime of pushing a car out of the mud.
2 Group form themselves together in preparation for mime, expressing strength in legs and lower body and shoulders and arms.
3 Group carry out the mime (in roles of either 'pushers' or 'car').
4 Group can release the strength at the point they choose, or imagine an ending (eg. the car not shifting; a sudden shift as it moves off; or a slow release as it is pushed on through and out of mud).

QUALITY 8

Aim: To develop quality of lightness
Population: All
Conditions: None
Time: 10 minutes
Equipment: Pieces of light material
Structure: Individual

■Activity

1   Leader distributes pieces of material.
2   Suggest group walk quietly without disturbing the material held by two corners in front/to side of body.
3   Moving in different directions with other movements, trying to retain material as still.
4   Throw the material and echo with body the way it falls to the floor.

DEVELOPMENT OF THEME

QUALITY 9

Aim: To develop quality of lightness
Population: All
Conditions: None
Time: 2–3 minutes
Equipment: None
Structure: Individual, pairs

■Activity

1 Leader suggests group move as though the air under their arms is sustaining them, as though gravity did not exist, like moon-walking.
2 In pairs, mime pumping the air into balloons under partner's arms. They then move as though lifted up and floating away. Partner then decides what happens next; for example, as though air was seeping out? as though the balloon had burst? Tell your partner what is to happen and they move in response.

DEVELOPMENT OF THEME

QUALITY 10

Aim: To develop quality of suddenness
Population: All
Conditions: None
Time: 3 minutes
Equipment: Wooden block or drum
Structure: Individual

■Activity

Group move hands and feet sharply in time to a tapping rhythm given by leader on block or drum.

QUALITY 11

Aim: To develop quality of lightness
Population: All
Conditions: None
Time: 2 minutes
Equipment: None
Structure: Whole group

■**Activity**

1   Group make circle, walk into centre as though on eggshells. Try not to break the shells.
2   Move out to edge of circle again and repeat, focusing on careful, light steps, air under arms, chest light.

QUALITY 12

Aim: To develop quality of sustained movement

Population: All

Conditions: None

Time: 2 minutes

Equipment: None

Structure: Individual

■Activity

1   Imagine a waterfall; the movement is continuous.
2   Move as though you are the water, in continual motion, whether as a trickle or rushing over boulders and cliffs.
3   Now move at half the speed.
4   Now, as though in slow-motion film, half as slow again.

■Additional outcome

Develops continuity of movement.

QUALITY 13

Aim: To develop quality of sustained movement

Population: All

Conditions: None

Time: 3 minutes

Equipment: None

Structure: Pairs

■Activity

1 Leader suggests each pair select a game together (eg. tennis).
2 Mime the game in slow motion.
3 Share with another pair, who have to guess the game.

CHINESE WHISPERS

Aim: To practise imitation skills

Population: Adolescents, adults

Conditions: None

Time: 5 minutes

Equipment: None

Structure: Whole group or several small groups

■Activity

1 Group in circle standing one behind the other.
2 Leader gives instructions that each person should imitate any movement, however slight, that they notice the person in front making. No-one, however, is to move purposefully, other than to imitate the person in front.
3 The leader makes one purposeful movement to begin the group movement. The person behind the leader repeats it so that the movement is passed around the circle.
4 Allow group to experience the movements which evolve from all the unconscious movement emitted from members.

■Additional outcome

Awareness of how much movement we generate without full consciousness.

See page 128 for this activity used in another stage.

DIRECTIONALITY 2

Aim: To create a self-initiated structure

Population: All

Conditions: None

Time: 4 minutes

Equipment: Music of their choice

Structure: Individual

■**Activity**

1   Leader suggests that participants find a space for themselves.

2   While in that space, travel forwards, backwards, sideways and turn in various combinations.

3   Select several directions and create a repeatable but simple sequence of movement with the music as an accompaniment.

DEVELOPMENT OF THEME

PLANES 1

Aims: To explore preferences and develop non-habitual movement pattern

Population: All

Conditions: None

Time: 5 minutes

Equipment: None

Structure: Individual, partners

■Activity

1 Rise and sink to and from the high level (*see Glossary*).

2 Open and close at the medium level.

3 Forward and backward rolls at the low level.

4 Explore the plane(s) that are the most difficult or unusual for you to move within.

5 Begin with movement in one of the 'easiest' planes and add on movement from step 4 above to make a growth sequence.

6 Think of a word to describe the transition from the 'easy' to the more difficult/unusual planes.

7 Share movement and word with a partner.

■Supplementary development of activity

Discussion of habits and patterns in movement preferences, reference to the transition phase when attempting change.

DEVELOPMENT OF THEME

PLANES 2

Aim: To provide clear phrasing from a rhythmical structure
Population: Children
Conditions: Warmed up, especially in feet and legs
Time: 3–4 minutes
Equipment: None
Structure: Individual

■Activity

1 Leader suggests a movement phrase such as 'jump, jump, jump, jump; turn, turn, turn; jump and turn, jump and turn, jump and turn'.
2 Leader then suggests participants make up own rhythms, using jump and turn.

■Additional outcome

Energises group.

TENSION–RELAXATION 3

Aims: To release tension, co-operation, change of tension

Population: Not known violent groups

Conditions: Safety rules reiterated

Time: 3–4 minutes

Equipment: Possibly percussion

Structure: Small groups

■Activity

1   In small groups, interpret a volcano exploding.
2   Build up tension slowly, using vocalisation if appropriate.
3   Explode outwards, move through imaginary stages of lava slowly
    flowing then solidifying like a rock formation (stillness).
4   Share each group's interpretation.
5   Do as a whole group.

PASS

Aim: To become aware of sound and movement in group
Population: All
Conditions: None
Time: 10 minutes
Equipment: Music
Structure: Group

■Activity

1 Pass a sound around circle.
2 Pass a movement around circle.
3 With music to accompany the group, they follow leader's movement until she says 'pass'; then next one on right develops that movement for a while. When they feel group is following it okay, they then say 'pass', and so on.

CLAP

Aims: To let go of control in group and allow the group to develop own structures

Population: All

Conditions: None

Time: 10 minutes

Equipment: None

Structure: Whole group

■Activity

1 Begin by telling group they will make a group rhythm through clapping, sound making and movement — a group improvisation (6 minutes).

2 Leader asks for people to indicate if they believe they are not rhythmical, suggests that this activity may show that they are.

3 Begin with each member making their own clapping sound at random, simultaneously, in the circle. Closing eyes sometimes helps overcome inhibitions.

4 Let the clapping stimulate 'stamping' movement across the centre of the circle, voice sounds etc. Leader may have to 'hold' the experience, participating and picking up on rhythms as they emerge.

5 Allow ending to be spontaneous.

DEVELOPMENT OF THEME

PERCUSSION

Aims: Impulse control, taking initiatives

Population: Children, adolescents

Conditions: None

Time: 15–25 minutes

Equipment: Variety of percussion instruments

Structure: Individual and two groups

■Activity

1 Participants asked to explore the sound their selected instrument makes. Leader to guide this.

2 As a group, can only move when an individual initiates a sound. Freeze if someone else then comes in with their sound.

3 Leader can say 'change' and/or call out names to play sounds for a while, then encourage individuals to take own initiative.

■Supplementary development of activity

1 Suggest one group become the orchestra and the other the movers. The sound then accompanies the movement (which could be rehearsed first for 5 minutes). Give 3 minutes for this. Change over roles.

2 Suggest they now use sound as the stimulus for the movement. Orchestra plays and the movers dance out the music. (NB. Movers need to be encouraged to interact as a group in the dance.)

■Additional outcomes

1 A self-initiated group choreography with own musical accompaniment.

2 Self-confidence in movement.

COLOURS 1

Aims: To work with colour in movement and explore our feelings in relation to colour

Population: All

Conditions: None

Time: 20–30 minutes

Equipment: None

Structure: Individual and group

■Activity

1 Leader suggests group move for 10 seconds to each of the following colours; red, green, blue, yellow, pink etc.
2 Ask group to call out own choices.
3 In pairs; one moves to a colour of their choice, the other guesses it.
4 Three groups; leader gives a colour to each group who then have one minute to rehearse its expression as a group, then perform it. Other groups guess the colour.
5 Each group thinks of own colour, rehearses and performs it for others to guess.

COLOURS 2

Aims: To work with colour in movement and explore our feelings in relation to colour

Population: All

Conditions: None

Time: 20–30 minutes

Equipment: Paper and felt-tip pens

Structure: Individual

■Activity

1 Close eyes; imagine colour yellow; you are moving in yellowness.
2 This gradually changes from a dark yellow to misty to white (give a couple of minutes in each shade).
3 Gradually visualise out of the white a colour that is soothing for you.
4 Bring it out, dance with it, play and enjoy it (3 minutes).
5 Say goodbye to the colour, knowing it is always there for you.
6 Draw your colour dance.
7 Share picture in large group feedback.

COLOURS 3

Aims: To work with colour in movement and explore our feelings in relation to colour

Population: All

Conditions: None

Time: 1 hour

Equipment: Paper and felt-tip pens

Structure: Individual and groups

■Activity

1   Select either red, yellow or green and make a picture of one of these colours (using all colours you like) to depict emotions and associations.

2   Walk round all pictures and write on slips of paper your associations and your guess of which colour it depicts. Put paper under picture.

3   Return to your own picture and put colour and association on piece of paper at top of picture.

4   Walk round all pictures again reading these.

5   Walk to next picture along from yours. Make a movement which expresses all of it or some aspect of it. Move to the next with that movement and do the same. If you meet anyone, interact with them as you go. Make it flow. This is a group dance of all your perceptions of these colours.

6   Return to your own picture, read the words underneath. Share in pairs what you have found and any connections between what your colour was expressing and others' perceptions.

7   Group sharing of dance pictures and thoughts.

■Supplementary development of activity

1   All 'reds', 'yellows' and 'greens' could meet and, using their pictures as guides, dance out the colour.

2   Share dance with other groups.

DARKNESS & LIGHT

Aim: To become aware of blind spots
Population: Adults
Conditions: Well-established group
Time: 20 minutes
Equipment: Paper and felt-tips
Structure: Individual

■Activity

1   Draw an image that is to do with darkness and light (4 minutes).
2   Using the picture as a map, move from the darkness to the light (4 minutes).
3   In fours or fives; select one aspect of the improvisation you would like to explore further with the group's support. Group will give help in movement and sound to enable that individual really to dance out that aspect.
4   Discuss in turn your feelings, memories, images and any other connections you may have made for yourself.

■Supplementary development of activity

Individual could repeat the dance with any new awareness.

WE ARE OUR BODIES 1

Aim: To sense our body image

Population: All

Conditions: When group is well established

Time: 1 hour

Equipment: Large roll of paper, felt-tip pens, paint, crayons

Structure: Individual, pairs, whole group

■Activity

1   In a group mingle together, meet each other in turn (leader says 'change') and say one thing about your body to partner, starting with the words 'I am . . .'.

2   Now repeat, but express one thing you notice about your partner's body.

3   Collect paper and cut it to the length you believe your body to be (do not measure it up against you first).

4   Meditation preparation (5 minutes); have them sit near their paper in a comfortable position, eyes closed if possible. Draw their attention to breath, floor, body in contact with itself and floor. Move on to talk about the 'sense of body self'. Ask them to reflect upon how they care for their bodies, clothe them, take part in physical activities; what about sexuality? Breathe deeply 5 times and open eyes.

5   Suggest they draw a portrait of their bodies on the paper (15 minutes).

6   Put the portrait up on the wall.

7   Stand back 5 or 6 feet and look at it. For 15 minutes, allow and receive the dance within you as it begins to move in response to the portrait. Follow the impulses to move.

8   Re-make the essence of that dance for 2 minutes. Draw it on a small sheet of paper, give it a title.

9   Turn portrait around towards wall.

10   In pairs, in turn, share essence of dance. Partner draws what he observes during/after dance. Give it a title. 2 minutes each, no talking.

11   Discuss in same pairs the similarities/differences in the drawing.

WE ARE OUR BODIES 2

Aim: To sense our body image

Population: All

Conditions: When group is well established   **Time:** 1 hour

Equipment: Large roll of paper, felt-tip pens, paint, crayons

Structure: Individual, pairs, whole group

■Activity

1 Take portrait and use marks to illustrate where non-functional areas are, eg. weakness, strengths, hot, cold, associations.

2 Mark your portrait with a colour, shape and quality that is expressive of these.

3 Select one mark and make a movement to symbolise it.

4 Allow the movement to become a sensation in that area of your body. Close eyes and take a few minutes to sense this area. Breathe slowly and deeply.

5 Let torso begin to move slightly to express the sensation.

6 Repeat several times, noticing the quality and shape of movement. Does the movement want to take you across the space? What is the rhythm? Are there any images appearing, sounds, words?

7 Remember the mark; does the movement still fit? Let it develop so you are able to express it clearly. Exaggerate its shape.

8 In fours, share main aspect of your 'mark dance'. Others give feedback in non-critical manner.

9 Performer takes 2 minutes to draw anything which comes to mind afterwards. Meanwhile next one is sharing their dance.

10 All complete sentence, 'my body is telling me . . .'

11 Share in large group the pictures and sentences.

12 Closure (individually): close eyes, suggest they breathe, and talk them through a grounding of body, ie in contact with the floor, how far from walls, door, back to the self.

■Supplementary development of activity

See *We Are Our Bodies 1.* Use that activity as a supplementary development to the above.

HAND DANCES

Aim: To become aware of self with another in movement

Population: All

Conditions: None

Time: 10 minutes

Equipment: Music (classical guitar)

Structure: Pairs

■Activity

1   In pairs, close eyes sitting opposite each other and make contact with left wrists.

2   Explore space between you while maintaining a protective space for yourself.

3   After 3–4 minutes have them stand up while maintaining the contact.

4   Now have them change wrists without losing contact.

5   Now have them travel forward/backwards/sideways. Who initiates? How does this affect your space?

6   After 10 minutes have them find a way to come to a resolution.

■Additional outcome

Awareness of personal space needs.

STILLNESS IN MOVEMENT

Aim: To enable group to become aware of group's theme(s) in movement

Population: Adolescents, adults

Conditions: None

Time: 5–10 minutes

Equipment: None

Structure: Whole group (minimum 3)

■Activity

1   Stand in a circle, one behind the other.
2   Simply watch the person in front of you and move in precisely the same way that they do (NB. No-one is to move consciously — shadow movements only.)

■Additional outcomes

1   Extension of normal movement range.
2   Awareness of group tension.

INTERPERSONAL

Aim: To become aware of self in relation to others

Population: Adults

Conditions: Long attention span required

Time: 45 minutes

Equipment: None

Structure: Individual

■Activity

1   Move with the sensation you feel in your body, eg. lightness, agility, resistance, heaviness. You are as if alone, encountering yourself moving.

2   Use familiar movements to make a pathway around the space.

3   Repeat patterning and movements so that you know them. There is a beginning, a middle and an end. Do not acknowledge or communicate with any people or objects. Maintain an inward frame of mind.

4   What are the bodily sensations you notice while on this journey? Enlarge these sensations and express them in movement.

5   Now repeat pathway 3 times and exaggerate your movements. Return to beginning of pathway, close eyes in that space and remember the path.

6   Now repeat pathway 3 times but notice other people/objects as you go. Who do you notice on your pathway? Continue your journey, being aware of any bodily sensations and movement, and if they change as you notice others. Who do you select to notice? Do not interact, just notice. Exaggerate those changes in body sensation as expressed in movement. Return to the beginning of your pathway, close eyes and replay the journey.

7   Now repeat the pathway 3 times, this time interacting with others. Who do you choose and who chooses you? Do you initiate or do they? Who leaves first? Notice your body sensations and movement. Exaggerate any changes you are aware of. Return to beginning of pathway and close eyes, remembering journey.

8   Again travel pathway 3 times but only noticing others. What/who do you notice? What is the body/movement like now; any differences? Exaggerate them. Return and remember.

9 Alone again, travel your pathway for the last time (3 times) and notice how the frame of mind manifests itself in your movement. Is it different from the last time you were alone on your pathway? Return and remember.

10 Take a sheet of paper with 5 columns, headed.

(a) 'when I am alone',
(b) 'when I notice',
(c) 'when I interact',
(d) 'when I notice again',
(e) 'when I'm alone again'.

Brainstorm for 1 minute per column anything you remember; words, sensations, movements, experience, actions, feelings, thoughts, images.

11 In pairs, discuss experiences from each column and relate to life events.

■Supplementary development of activity

1 Before any discussion in pairs, you could select one word from each column and share it in hand gesture. Do not let your partner see the words. Make hands express sensation, etc.

2 Partner (a) guesses the word; (b) replies in hand gesture using their selection of words from same columns.

3 Interact together in hand dance, using any of the selected words as starting-points. Keep to movement repertoire already experienced.

4 Complete the following sentence individually: 'My body tells me . . .'

5 Select one of the columns and draw a picture that expresses it.

6 Large group discussion and sharing of picture.

SHAPING SPACE .

Aim: To explore the relationship you have with space, and it with you

Population: Any experienced movement group

Conditions: None

Time: 10–15 minutes

Equipment: None

Structure: Individual

■Activity

1 Move as though in a space that is
   - (a) tight,
   - (b) narrow,
   - (c) convex,
   - (d) concave,
   - (e) overhanging,
   - (f) steep,
   - (g) towering,
   - (h) very expansive (eg. a plain).

2 Using the expansive space as a starting-point, guide movers from the grassy plain into the air, up and away from the land to the heavens and outer space.

3 Guide them into a 'planet dance' which takes place in Father Sky but returns to Mother Earth in a group, and let them sway together.

4 Finish with a grounding (*see Glossary*) or centring (*see Glossary*) of the group. For example, sitting cross-legged, being aware of spine, seat bones and breath.

5 Discuss the 'planet dance' as a group.

■Supplementary development of activity

1 Select one aspect of your experience of moving in space and make a picture of it (5 minutes). Give the picture a title.

2 In threes; one moves to express their picture and others share what it felt like to watch them (no critical comments).

LINES 2

Aim: To interact with partner
Population: All
Conditions: Early sessions
Time: 10 minutes
Equipment: Paper and felt-tips
Structure: Pairs

■Activity

1 Make markings on the paper together and explore qualities of line.
2 Now, with a clean sheet of paper, use marking of lines to interact in a line conversation.
3 Use the drawing as a map for having a movement conversation together.

■Supplementary development of activity

5 minutes to reflect upon the experience and state what was appreciated and resented about the last interaction.

■Additional outcome

Awareness of what we say to each other using non-verbal media only.

DEVELOPMENT OF THEME

RELATIONSHIP 5

Aims: To observe and respond to another in movement
Population: Adolescents, adults
Conditions: Some improvisation skills
Time: 3–5 minutes
Equipment: Music of choice
Structure: Pairs

■Activity

1   With a partner, mirror or contrast movements and have a movement conversation or argument (30 seconds).
2   What were the words or phrases that could describe the experience (discuss for 1 minute)?
3   Repeat conversation, allowing words to accompany movement.
4   In what ways do you normally enhance your communication (words and movement)? Ask for feedback from partner.

■Additional outcomes

Insights into mismatching of words and movement in communication. How misunderstandings can arise in the 'reading' of body movement. Awareness of authentic movement supporting words.

DEVELOPMENT OF THEME

RELATIONSHIP 6

Aim: To develop leadership qualities
Population: All
Conditions: None
Time: 2–3 minutes
Equipment: None
Structure: One or two groups and volunteer

■Activity

1   One member volunteers to conduct the group, using hands, giving non-verbal signals to promote a movement activity (for example, arms up and down quickly to promote jumping).

2   Discuss the group's interpretation of the signals.

■Supplementary development of activity

Conduct two groups simultaneously, using left and right hands to give signals.

RELATIONSHIP 7

Aims: To encourage meeting and parting

Population: Children and adolescents

Conditions: When maintaining relationships is difficult. Ensure safety rules (not to let go of elastic)

Time: 2–3 minutes

Equipment: Elastic, 1–2 inches wide, 5–6 feet long, hand hole securely sewn in each end
Plenty of space

Structure: Pairs

■Activity

1   Using the elastic to link partners, suggest a moving apart and running together so they pass each other.
2   Vary side of body passed (eg. right sides and left sides).
3   As they run towards each other, elastic shrinks, then stretches as they part again, allowing for tension which encourages a recoil again for a return to the meeting place.

■Supplementary development of activity

Perhaps make noise as they run.

■Additional outcomes

1   Tension-relaxation.
2   Separation, yet linked in relationship.
3   Co-operation.

RELATIONSHIP 8

Aim: To relate to objects
Population: All
Conditions: Confidence in improvisation
Time: About 2 minutes
Equipment: Any appropriate prop
Structure: Individual

■Activity

1 Approach and make contact with the prop.
2 Explore it in movement.
3 Move with it for 40 seconds.
4 Leave the prop.

■Supplementary development of activity

1 Discuss the qualities of the prop in pairs.
2 Share your 40 seconds dance with your partner.

RELATIONSHIP 9

Aim: To express anger
Population: Adolescents
Conditions: Safety rules reiterated, small group
Time: 1–2 minutes
Equipment: Soft beach balls, large wall space (no windows)
Structure: Individual

■Activity

1   Each member faces the wall area (well defined) and throws the ball hard against it.
2   Repeat for 1 minute, encourage use of sound as they throw.
3   Suggest they use words such as 'I hate . . .'.
4   Discuss in group.

DEVELOPMENT OF THEME

RELATIONSHIP 10

Aims: Structuring and channelling energy
Population: All
Conditions: Safety structures
Time: Variable
Equipment: Mats/cushions
Structure: Whole group

■Activity

1   Slap or bang hands on a mat/cushion with clear phrasing (eg. bang, bang, BANG) then no pushing.
2   Leader to maintain leadership role in channelling energy towards a resolution.

RELATIONSHIP 11

Aims: To identify and communicate needs
Population: All
Conditions: Able to work in small group alone
Time: 5–10 minutes
Equipment: None
Structure: Small groups of 3 or 4

■Activity

1 Each member in turn asks group to do something for them, eg. give them a swing, jump them high, a rock, a trust fall, etc.
2 Leader may have previously given opportunities for various small group activities; individuals select one they would especially like for themselves.
3 Leader must be conscious of over-ambitious groups, for example, with regard to carrying, catching and ensuring safety aspects are adhered to (how to carry, hold safely another human being).

■Supplementary development of activity

1 Perhaps then engage whole group in doing something for someone.
2 Leader could ask group to give them a rock or ride of some sort.

RELATIONSHIP 12

Aim: Nurturing a partner
Population: All
Conditions: None
Time: 5–6 minutes
Equipment: Mats
Structure: Threes

■Activity

1 Two kneel down opposite each other; the third lies between them and is rolled carefully from one set of knees across to the other.

2 Change roles so all have a turn in the middle.

RELATIONSHIP 13

Aims: Trust and letting go
Population: All
Conditions: None
Time: Variable
Equipment: None
Structure: Threes

■Activity

1   In threes, standing, two catchers face each other with the third, who is to be pivoted and rocked back and forth between them, in the middle.

2   Distance between the two catchers depends on the group's needs, but begin fairly close so there is not too far for the middle one to fall.

3   Middle one remains rigid, like a metal rod, and is passive. Catchers use wide stance, knees bent and hands wide open to receive weight. Contact shoulder blades and upper chest.

4   Change roles.

■Supplementary development of activity

Middle one decides when to rock back and forth, taking an active role.

DIRECTIONALITY 3

Aim: To experience the backward direction (into the unknown)

Population: All (must have some ego)

Conditions: Emphasis on safety ground rules

Time: 10–35 minutes

Equipment: None

Structure: Individually and partners

■Activity

1 Individually walk backwards from one side of space to other. Slowly move with eyes fixed on object in front, be aware of distance increasing as journey continues into the unknown — the future — back to the future.

2 In pairs; roles of 'wise guide' (super ego) and 'journeyer'. Wise guide supports partner as they move backwards by standing in front and using voice and/or touch to help them on their journey.

3 Next have participants put out chairs and other objects in the space. Repeat journey, the partner acting as guide.

4 Repeat journey with guide behind journeyer (if contact is made with others by journeyer, help journeyer to explore these others gently).

5 Change roles.

■Supplementary development of activity

1 Repeat each section 1–5 above, but journeyer closes eyes.

2 Could also repeat each section 2–5 but without 'wise guide'. Each participant is a combination of wise guide and journeyer.

■Additional outcomes

1 Development of giving and receiving support/guidance from others.

2 Brings out the theme of the unknown, fear in exploration.

3 Encourages change of pace for underbounded (*see Glossary*) groups.

4 Promotes sense of a base, and moving out from there to explore environment.

5 Can act as an integrator of the actor and observer roles.

DEVELOPMENT OF THEME

BODY BOUNDARY 3

Aims: To give and receive peer attention, to develop trust, sensitivity and awareness of self affecting others

Population: Adolescents and adults

Conditions: Safety rules

Time: 10 minutes

Equipment: None

Structure: Partners in whole group

■Activity

1 All stand in a circle.
2 Pummel all soft areas of own body and chest (making sound).
3 Turn to person (partner) on left and pummel with loose fists the other's calves, thighs, buttocks, backs, shoulders, upper arms.
4 Finish by stroking from the top of their head down to their feet slowly in one gentle sweep.
5 Turn to your right and repeat with that person.
6 Notice the differences in contact between the two people massaging you.
7 Notice your responses to them and any differences.

■Supplementary development of activity

1 After the above, open up a large group discussion which encourages each person to give feedback to those who massaged them.
2 Ask how it felt to be getting and giving this kind of attention from each other.

■Additional outcomes

A recognition of the part physical contact plays in their lives. A new level of relationship with peers. The ability to give and receive feedback from peers. Giving and receiving attention in a group.

See page 134 for this activity used in another stage.

BODY BOUNDARY 6

Aim: To let go enough to experience self and others
Population: Adults
Conditions: Middle to end of sessions
Time: 5 minutes
Equipment: None
Structure: Individual, pairs

■Activity

1 Give yourself a hug while sitting down.
2 Repeat standing.
3 Give another group member a hug in the same manner as you gave yourself one.
4 Tell them how you experienced their hug.
5 Any ideas about how you took care of yourself?

■Supplementary development of activity

Hug each member of the group in turn.

■Additional outcomes

An increased sense of self. Through this physical contact some issues may arise concerning their experience of being held or touched when an infant/child. There may be an opening up to self-care and to caring for others.

See page 243 for this activity used in another stage.

BODY BOUNDARY 7

Aims: To experience being moved and receiving that experience from others; to be in a moving relationship without any direct physical contact; to establish sense of self as separate from the environment

Population: All, particularly young children

Conditions: Before introducing touch

Time: 10 minutes

Equipment: Large pieces of strong material

Structure: Pairs, small groups

■Activity

1   In pairs, one partner (volunteer) is wrapped in the material.
2   Partner spins, pulls and swings them, slowly at first.
3   Reverse roles of activator and volunteer and repeat.
4   Form small groups; give a volunteer a ride across the floor in the material.

■Supplementary development of activity

1   Find a beginning, middle and end for the group process. Share your story with the whole group.
2   First volunteers, then activators, give comments to whole group.

■Additional outcomes

Sense of being in receipt of a moving experience generated by peer(s). Sense of body, since in contact with the floor through the material. Free-flowing exercise.

BODY BOUNDARY 8

Aim: To encourage sense of self and others through whole bodily contact

Population: Adults and children

Conditions: After some physical contact has been introduced

Time: 15 minutes

Equipment: None

Structure: Pairs, whole group

■Activity

1 Partners grip wrist to wrist as one slides partner across floor on their back. Give time for trust to build.
2 Ensure they feel their waist by wriggling the sliding partner.
3 Reverse roles.
4 Now both take up a long stretched rolling movement together, with hand to hand contact.
5 Practise rolling from one end of the space to the other in pairs.
6 Whole group positioned side by side prone on floor, partners head to head.
7 In turn, each pair roll over the whole group, trying to keep hands linked and rolling at the same time. Ensure no spaces between people on floor.

■Supplementary development of activity

1 Slide partners towards a people pile in the centre of the space.
2 Roll together into a people pile. Ensure people are in contact with each other both during the making of the pile and at the finish.
3 Take a couple of minutes to relax as a whole group on each other's bodies.
4 Slowly roll away from each other into a space on your own. Notice the contact with the floor as opposed to people.

■Additional outcomes

Development of group cohesion. Sense of self as separate from others. Active-passive experience.

BALANCE 7

Aims: Inner control, accepting a structure
Population: Children
Conditions: None
Time: 5 minutes
Equipment: None
Structure: Individual, pairs, small groups

■Activity

1 Leader gives a balance position which is held by all participants; eg. two hands and one foot, seat, shoulders.
2 After, say, 5 seconds another balance is given.
3 Gradually make the balances more difficult, eg. decrease the surface area in contact with the floor.
4 Repeat with a partner who is teaming up to make the given balance. Encourage physical contact.
5 Change partners on each balance.
6 Repeat in small groups.

■Supplementary development of activity

1 Repeat whole exercise within a confined space, eg. on a mat.
2 Travel in the balance to other end of room.

■Additional outcomes

Can restrict impulsive action and act as a containment for hyperactivity. Working with others to a given structure, problem solving.

PERSONAL SPACE 6

Aim: Awareness of object world in relation to self
Population: All
Conditions: None
Time: 5 minutes
Equipment: Ball, mat, chair, bean bag, hoop
Structure: Individual

■Activity

1 Place an object near to participant. Suggest they focus on object.
2 Suggest they move towards the object; ensure they are close but not touching the object.
3 Suggest they explore moving around it at first.
4 Develop the exploration by suggesting movement over, to one side, other side, in front of and behind the object at various distances but where they could still reach the object if need be.

■Supplementary development of activity

1 Reach for, touch and grasp the object, integrating it into closer proximity of body exploring relationships in space with the object.
2 Grasp and let go of the object in personal space while remaining glued to one spot.
3 In twos, explore the object in own personal space; how it can be moved, related to, etc. Stay rooted to one place on floor. When the object is released by design or accident out of the place, the partner retrieves and continues exploration for themselves in the same manner in own personal space.
4 Leader could stipulate 30 seconds or 1 minute per person before change-over; could accompany with light piano music.

■Additional outcomes

An awareness of objects in relation to manipulation skills within own space. Development of exploratory senses towards:
(a) moving an object in relation to the body and spaces created by the body
(b) moving the body in relation to a still object.

PERSONAL SPACE 7
(Slow Motion Boxing)

Aims: To move in and out of personal space

Population: Adolescents, particularly boys

Conditions: None

Time: 5 minutes

Equipment: Mats and sustained musical accompaniment

Structure: Pairs

■Activity

1 Each pair on a mat, or in designated space, kneeling down facing each other. Leader suggests that a movement dialogue will take place between them for 30 seconds where no touching is allowed. The game is called 'slow motion boxing' and the idea is that one initiates a movement towards the other who responds by pulling away, then miming a movement back.

2 Falling sideways, backwards as a response can be encouraged.

3 Only allow, for example, four punches each to ensure that the slow motion element is adhered to.

4 They must contain the movement dialogue to the confined space (eg. the mat).

■Supplementary development of activity

1 Repeat half-kneeling.

2 Repeat standing.

3 Discussion could centre on control of fighting impulses, play fighting.

4 Teach 'how to fall' onto the floor.

■Additional outcomes

Some awareness of body control, how to fall, and the relationship of mind to body in aggression.

BODY INVENTORY

Aims: To promote bodily and social awareness

Population: Children, adults

Conditions: Once trust and group cohesion are established

Time: 10 minutes

Equipment: None

Structure: Individual, partner, group

■Activity

Leader calls out two body parts, eg. ear to knee. Either part is moved towards the other part until they are in contact.

■Supplementary development of activity

1 Have the individual travel with parts in contact.
2 Have people contact another person, part to part.
3 Have the whole group in physical contact and perform a task such as sitting, swaying, jumping without losing contact.
4 Could use same parts, eg. feet to feet.

■Additional outcomes

The group should begin to focus on and identify different body parts. The physical contact with others can enable a different sort of closeness in the group to emerge. Often laughter results from, say, travelling with parts in contact.

RELAXATION

Aim: To be aware of own body
Population: All except children
Conditions: None
Time: 10 minutes
Equipment: None
Structure: Individual

■**Activity**

1   In a quiet room with softened lighting, lie on back, become aware of breathing.
2   Take in a few deep breaths and, while exhaling, mentally say the word 'relax'.
3   Concentrate on face and feel any tension in eyes and face. Let it relax and become comfortable, like a tight rubber band going limp. Feel this wave of relaxation through whole body.
4   Tense the eyes and face, grit teeth and then relax and feel it spread through body as a whole.
5   Repeat 4 for each body part, moving from neck down to toes. Picture in mind tension and it melting away.
6   Rest for 2–5 minutes afterwards.
7   Let muscles and eyelids lighten up and become ready to open eyes, become aware of room.
8   Let eyes open and be ready to stand up.

PUSHING

Aims: To channel aggression, get a sense of own power

Population: All

Conditions: No violence

Time: 5 minutes

Equipment: None

Structure: Pairs

■Activity

1 In pairs, push against each other, back to back, while sitting. Leader to count '5,4,3,2,1' for time allowed. Aim to push partner across floor.
2 Change partners.
3 Change to pushing hips to hips, shoulders to shoulders and hands to hands, in that order, each with a different partner.

■Supplementary development of activity

1 One partner says 'yes' and one 'no' during the activity (pairs decide who says which).
2 Reflection upon what the conflict was like, which role you chose to play, etc.

■Additional outcomes

1 Assertion.
2 Development of quality of strength and bound flow (*see Laban movement analysis*).

CO-OPERATION

Aim: To work together when touch is not appropriate

Population: All

Conditions: Safety

Time: 5 minutes

Equipment: Light garden sticks or canes; music if preferred

Structure: Pairs

■Activity

1 In pairs, each take hold of one end of the stick lightly in fingers.
2 Each leading and following, explore where and how the stick can move. Explore the space between each other. Do not allow the stick to fall.

■Supplementary development of activity

Develop to using two sticks.

■Additional outcomes

1 Development of restraining flow focused in the space.
2 Development of sensitivity and sense of lightness.

CARRY

Aims: To support one another in the group, teach lifting strategies

Population: All

Conditions: Trust

Time: 10–15 minutes

Equipment: Possibly a large, strong piece of material for lifters to hold person in

Structure: Groups of five, seven or nine

■Activity

1 In groups; each group supports fully the weight of one member. Lifters ensure hands are under person's shoulders, hips, head and knees; lifters link arms and bend knees.

2 Progress to carrying the member around the room.

3 Progress to lifting them above heads.

■Supplementary development of activity

1 Lifters could use material for carrying.

2 Progress to swaying or swinging each member.

3 As a group, give a ride to the person by pulling them along the floor in the material.

■Additional outcomes

1 Co-operation.

2 Letting go in a group.

3 Trust.

BODY CONTROL 7

Aims: To reduce impulsivity and promote spatial co-ordination

Population: Children, adults

Conditions: None

Time: 2 minutes

Equipment: None

Structure: Whole group

■Activity

1   Suggest the group walk very fast around the edge of the space in the same direction.
2   Ask them to spiral slowly inwards until centre of space is reached, coming to a stop on arrival.
3   Gradually spiral out again.
4   Repeat inwards spiral and finish in cluster at centre in stillness, then face the walls and walk away from group.
5   Repeat 1–4, but running instead of walking.

■Additional outcomes

Working as a group in movement and space.

BODY CONTROL 8

Aims: Physical control and development of strength

Population: All

Conditions: None

Time: 2–3 minutes

Equipment: Rhythmical music

Structure: Individual

■Activity

1   Group copy leader demonstrating raising one leg slowly in standing position (use chair if required at first).

2   Change directions of leg raise, eg. forward, to one side, behind.

3   Repeat in prone position.

LEVEL 4

Aims: To promote wider vocabulary of movement and adaptation of movements to different levels (*see Glossary*)

Population: Children

Conditions: None

Time: 2–3 minutes

Equipment: None

Structure: Individually

■Activity

1 Leader suggests the upper part of the body is opened and stretched at a specific level (*see Glossary*); for example, stretching out arms horizontally while standing would be a stretch at the medium level.

2 Repeat this opening movement with the upper body but at another level; for example, the same stretch as above while lying down.

3 Now close and curl the upper part of the body at a specified level.

4 Repeat this closing movement at another level.

■Supplementary development of activity

1 Close upper and open lower part of the body, each at different levels, for example twist and hug the upper body while standing with feet wide apart.

2 Open upper and close lower part of the body, each at different levels.

■Additional outcome

Co-ordination between upper and lower parts of the body.

See page 167 for this activity used in another stage.

TENSION–RELAXATION 4

Aims: To reduce impulsivity and increase control

Population: All

Conditions: None

Time: 5–10 minutes

Equipment: Drum

Structure: Whole group

■Activity

1   Leader suggests they make a fist, clenching it to the count of 1–5.

2   Reverse count for release of fist and relaxation.

3   Shake out hand and arm.

4   Repeat on other side.

■Supplementary development of activity

1   Repeat above to drum beats (increase and decrease intensity of sound).

2   Repeat with the jaw area and other muscle groups.

■Additional outcome

Isolation of areas of body.

TENSION–RELAXATION 5

Aims: To relax group and separate for closure

Population: All

Conditions: None

Time: 4 minutes

Equipment: None

Structure: Individual

■Activity

1   All lying on backs on mats.

2   Suggest they close eyes and allow body to sink into floor heavily. Picture a blank white screen.

3   Imagine the sun warmly relaxing body, and the floor softly receiving body's weight.

4   Breathe out slowly four times; roll onto left side and wait. Open eyes slowly. Get up in own time.

TENSION–RELAXATION 6

Aim: To close group in manner whereby each is able to leave as an individual

Population: All

Conditions: None

Time: 2 minutes

Equipment: None

Structure: Individual

■**Activity**

1   Lie on floor with legs vertically against wall. Ensure base of spine is close to base of wall.

2   Slowly allow legs to open with their own weight, arms behind head.

3   Stay there and be aware of breath for 30 seconds or so.

4   Gently bring legs together, roll onto side and stand up.

■**Additional outcomes**

Endurance, inner body sensation, letting go, self-limits, self-trust.

TENSION–RELAXATION 7

Aims: To control and release muscle groups to promote relaxation

Population: All

Conditions: None

Time: 5–10 minutes

Equipment: Mats

Structure: Individual

■Activity

1 Group lie on backs on mats with open postures.
2 Leader suggests they close eyes, breathe out slowly three times, and respond to suggestions to tighten and relax muscles.
3 Go through areas of body from head to feet, suggesting main muscle groups (and smaller muscle groups if desired).
4 Leader selects participant's head, legs and arms to lift and test on a scale of tension–relaxation.

TENSION–RELAXATION 8

Aim: To close the group
Population: All
Conditions: None
Time: Open-ended
Equipment: None
Structure: Individual

■Activity

1   Lean back against wall in a sitting position on an imaginary seat.
2   Hold position, using tension in thighs, legs, abdominals.
3   See how long the position can be sustained.
4   Move away slowly from wall and shake out legs.

■Additional outcomes

Endurance, inner body sensation, self-limits.

TENSION–RELAXATION 9

Aim: To close the group
Population: All
Conditions: None
Time: 2 minutes
Equipment: None
Structure: Individual

■Activity

1   Move like a puppet on a string.
2   Move as though held and then flop as if dropped.
3   Move as though held again.

TENSION–RELAXATION 10

Aim: To close the group
Population: All
Conditions: None
Time: 2 minutes
Equipment: None
Structure: Whole group

■**Activity**

1 Spread fingers of one hand wide and then relax them.
2 Repeat with both hands.
3 Repeat with alternate hands.

FLOOR PATTERN 2

Aims: To experience leading and following as a linked group

Population: Adults, children

Conditions: None

Time: 3–4 minutes

Equipment: None

Structure: Whole group

■Activity

1 The group make a line holding hands. Designate one of the people on the end as leader.

2 For one minute they walk, twisting and coiling like a snake, following the leader around the space.

3 Reverse this sequence of movements as near as possible, following the person at the other end of line as the leader.

4 Repeat with a new leader and a different method of travel, for example zigzagging.

5 Ask for a volunteer, who then separates from the group.

6 The group continue but make their line into a knot, travelling around and under each other; when thoroughly knotted they freeze, but at no time unclasp hands.

7 The volunteer then attempts to untie the knot by physically manoeuvring the group.

■Supplementary development of activity

1 Volunteer undoes knot by giving verbal instructions only to group.

2 Group undo own knot non-verbally.

■Additional outcome

Physical contact is engendered.

See page 87 for this activity used in another stage.

BODY SENSATION 2

Aims: To become more aware of the tension in our bodies; to begin to release tension

Population: All

Conditions: None

Time: 5 minutes

Equipment: Drum

Structure: Individual

■Activity

1   While lying on the floor in open position, let eyes close.
2   Leader talks through a count of 1 to 5, during which each member tenses their whole body, including face, and holds breath.
3   Count down from 5 to 1 and release tension built up.
4   Count down from 5 to 1 again for further release using breath.
5   Repeat the above for specific body parts identified by group member.

■Supplementary development of activity

1   Use drum for build-up of tension; build up slowly in a crescendo.
2   Tension could be expressed in contraction, extension or twisting of body.

■Additional outcomes

Sense of the tension required and of excessive habitual tension which needs release. Quiet time can enable deep awareness of body.

See page 73 for this activity used in another stage.

MASSAGE

Aims: To warm self and group; relaxation of muscles after physical exertion

Population: All

Conditions: None

Time: 5–10 minutes

Equipment: None

Structure: Whole group

■Activity

1 Make a close circle, sitting or standing; one behind gently massages the shoulders of one in front.

2 Turn around and repeat.

3 Each to give feedback on how soft/hard they want massage.

See page 97 for this activity used in another stage.

STRETCH 1

Aims: To identify and move body parts and muscle groups
Population: All
Conditions: Each session
Time: 5 minutes
Equipment: Music or percussion
Structure: Individual, pairs

■Activity

1   Leader verbally identifies body parts in turn, and encourages a gradual stretch and release for each named part.
2   Change the levels for stretching, eg. lying, sitting.
3   Use accompaniment if desired.

■Supplementary development of activity

Partner B stretches A's limbs gently while lying on floor.

■Additional outcomes

Awareness of sensation and articulation in body.

See page 95 for this activity used in another stage.

GROUP MOVEMENT

Aim: To let go of left-overs and session work
Population: All
Conditions: Ending a session quietly
Time: 5 minutes
Equipment: Music
Structure: Whole group

■Activity

1 Standing in a circle, in turn lead a movement and say which part you are moving (or leader can specify).
2 Next person in circle moves with a movement that follows on logically.
3 Continue until all group have led movement.

RELATIONSHIP 14

Aim: To wait for turn
Population: All
Conditions: None
Time: Variable
Equipment: None
Structure: Whole group

■Activity

Chinese whispers with specific actions (eg. pass on the squeeze) suggested by leader. Action goes around a circle/down a line until it reaches leader again.

RELATIONSHIP 15

Aims: To ground and care for one another in the group

Population: All

Conditions: None

Time: 3–6 minutes

Equipment: Soft music

Structure: Pairs

■Activity

1   Sitting in pairs, one cradles partner in arms and legs and gives a caring rock.

2   Change over.

■Additional outcomes

Caring and sensitivity towards others.

BODY BOUNDARY 9

Aim: Differentiation from the environment
Population: All
Conditions: None
Time: 5 minutes
Equipment: None
Structure: Individual

■Activity

1 All lying relaxed on the floor, prone.
2 Press a named body part which is in contact with the floor down further towards the floor.
3 Use breath; on outbreath make the small movement towards the floor.
4 Work systematically through the whole body.
5 Finish with a slow whole body roll.
6 Notice the body in contact with the floor in the roll.
7 Find a way of standing, being aware of the parts as they leave contact with the floor and those that remain in contact.

■Supplementary development of activity

1 Press parts against each other, eg. hand to hand.
2 Press parts against a wall.
3 Press parts against a partner.

■Additional outcomes

Awareness of own limits, grounding the energy, relationship of body self to the environment.

BODY BOUNDARY 6

Aim: To let go enough to experience self and others
Population: Adults
Conditions: Middle to end of sessions
Time: 5 minutes
Equipment: None
Structure: Individual, pairs

■Activity

1   Give yourself a hug while sitting down.
2   Repeat standing.
3   Give another group member a hug in the same manner as you gave yourself one.
4   Tell them how you experienced their hug.
5   Any ideas about how you took care of yourself?

■Supplementary development of activity

Hug each member of the group in turn.

■Additional outcomes

An increased sense of self. Through this physical contact some issues may arise concerning their experiences of being held or touched when an infant/child. There may be an opening up to self-care and to caring for others.

See page 215 for this activity used in another stage.

BREATH 7

Aim: To focus on exhalation in one part of body

Population: All

Conditions: None

Time: 4–5 minutes

Equipment: None

Structure: Pairs

■Activity

1   Find a partner.

2   One sits with eyes closed and focuses on breathing out into the open hand of the partner.

3   Their partner places open hand on different areas of abdomen, chest, sides, back and when they feel the breath movement into their hand changes positioning to a different area on upper body.

4   Reverse roles.

■Additional outcomes

1   Quietening and focusing.

2   Sensitivity towards partner's touch.

BREATH 8

Aim: To promote sense of control
Population: All
Conditions: None
Time: 1–2 minutes
Equipment: None
Structure: Individuals

■Activity

1 In a circle, sitting, hold one nostril closed and breathe in and out through the other, slowly.
2 Reverse, other nostril held.

SECTION 4

INFORMATION

TRAINING IN DANCE MOVEMENT THERAPY

The essence of Dance Movement Therapy (DMT) lies in the process rather than the technique. How it is used will depend on your talents in the art of movement and dance as well as the receptivity of the client to dance and movement. It is crucial that you have the ability to attend, hear and listen to the client's communications in the dance or movement as well as to verbalisaitons.

If you are interested in developing your talents in dance and movement and in responding in depth to clients in this medium as a dance movement therapist, then a professional training course is imperative. Anyone who is working with groups is qualified in one of the helping professions, and/or has extended training or experience in dance and movement could consider entering the field as a professional practitioner.

There is one university based course currently available in the UK. This is a recognised 2-year part-time, 1-year full-time, Post Graduate Diploma in Dance Movement Therapy. For details write to:

The Arts Therapies Division
School of Art & Design
The University of Hertfordshire
Hatfield Campus, College Lane
Hatfield
Herts AL10 9AB
Tel 01707 284800
www.herts.ac.uk

There are other types of training at various levels, non-validated and validated by various bodies, and self-financing, available in the UK and abroad. For example:

The Laban Centre for Movement and Dance, Laurie Grove, New Cross, London SE14 6NH. (www.laban.co.uk).

Roehampton Institute, Roehampton Lane, London SW15 5PJ. (www.roehampton.ac.uk) Two-year part-time course (Froebel College).

Continuing Education at Hunter College, 695 Park Avenue, East Building, 10th Floor, New York, NY10021, USA. MS and MSW in Movement Therapy.

Antioch New England Graduate School, 40 Avon Street, Keene, NH 03431-13516, USA. (www.antioch.edu) MA in Dance Movement Therapy.

Pratt Institute, 200 Willoughby Avenue, Brooklyn, New York, NY 11205, USA. MA in Dance Movement Therapy.

UCLA, 405 Hilgard Avenue, Box 951361, Los Angeles, California 90024-1361, USA. MA in Dance Movement Therapy.

Hahnemann University, Broad & Vine, Mail Stop 472, Philadelphia, PA 19102-1192, USA. MA in Dance Movement Therapy.

HELPFUL ADDRESSES

The American Dance Therapy Association (ADTA), Suite 108, 2000 Century Plaza, 10632 Little Patuxent Parkway, Columbia, Maryland 21044, USA.

Art Therapy Italiana (www.arttherapy.it). Summer schools in Italy and a four-year dance therapy training in Italy, with Summer intensive.

The Association for Dance Movement Therapy (ADMT), c/o Quaker Meeting House, Wedmore Vale, Bristol BS3 5HX. Publishes quarterly newsletter, organises monthly workshops and Summer schools, publications, support groups, network.

Association for Humanistic Psychology, Westwood, 5 The Breeches, West Didsbury, Mancester M20 2BG.

Association for Humanistic Psychology Practitioners (AHPP), Therapy (register of accredited practitioners). Tel 0845 766 0236.

Association of Jungian Analysts, Flat 3, No 7 Eton Avenue, London NW3 3EL. Therapy and training.

Association of Professional Music Therapists, c/o The Administrator, 26 Hamlyn Road, Glastonbury, Somerset BA6 8HT.

Bonnie Bainbridge-Cohen, School for Body-Mind Centering, 189 Pondview Drive, Amherst, MA 01002-3230, USA. Certification course in Body-Mind Centering.

British Association of Art Therapists, Mary Ward House, 5 Tavistock Place, London WC1H 9SN.

British Association of Dramatherapists, 30c Bank Street, Kincardine, Fife, Scotland FR10 6LY.

British Association of Psychotherapists, 37 Mapesbury Road, London NW2 4HJ. Therapy and training.

Chiron Centre for Holistic Psychotherapy, 26 Eaton Rise, Ealing, London W5 2ER. Training and supervision.

Chisenhale Dance Space, 64–86 Chisenhale Road, London E3 5QZ. Range of dance and movement courses.

Dance Books Ltd, The Old Bakery, 4 Lenten Street, Alton, Hampshire GU34 1HG. Stocks DMT titles.

Dance Movement Therapy Consultancy: supervision, groups and individual therapy practice. Helen Payne, 1 The Wick, High Street, Kimpton, Herts SG4 8SA. Tel 01438 833440.

Gestalt Centre, 62 Paul Street, London EC2A 4NA (www.gestaltcentre.co.uk). Training in Gestalt therapy. Supervision.

Guild of Psychotherapists, 47 Nelson Square, London SE1 0ZA.

Institute for the Arts in Psychotherapy, 1 Beaconsfield Road, St Albans, Herts AL1 3RD. Therapy/workshops. Tel 01438 833440.

University of Hertfordshire, Arts Therapies Division, Hatfield Campus, College Lane, Hatfield, Herts AL10 9AB. Organises Easter and Summer schools, weekend courses in DMT. PG Diploma in DMT.

Institute of Group Analysis, 1 Daleham Gardens, London NW3 5BY. Training and therapy.

Laban Guild, Mrs Ann Ward, 30 Ringsend Road, Limavady, Co. Derry BT49 0QL. Workshops in the Laban approach.

Lincoln Clinic and Institute for Psychotherapy, 77 Westminster Bridge Road, London SE1 7HS. Training and therapy.

London Association for Primal Psychotherapists, West Hill House, 6 Swains Lane, London N6 6QS.

London Centre for Psychotherapy, 32 Leighton Road, Kentish Town, London NW5 2QE. Training and supervision.

London Contemporary Dance School, The Place, 17 Dukes Road, London WC1H 9PY. Variety of courses.

Metanoia, Psychotherapy Training Institute, 13 North Common Road, Ealing, London NW5 2QB. Supervision and training.

National Resource Centre for Dance, University of Surrey, Guildford, Surrey GU2 7XH.

Post Reichian Therapy Association (Energy Stream), 23 Knowle Road, Leeds 4. Training and therapy.

Psychosynthesis and Education Trust, Tooley Street, London SE1 2TH.

Scottish Institute for Human Relations, 21 Elmbank Street, Glasgow G2 4PE. Training.

Shape, 7 Fitzroy Square, London W1P 6AE (arts opportunities for people with disabilities).

The Society of Analytical Psychotherapists, 1 Daleham Gardens, London NW3 5BY. Therapy.

Society for Dance Research, Laban Centre London, Laurie Grove, New Cross, London SE14 6NH.

Spectrum, 7 Endymion Road, London N41 4EE. Anatomy and Physiology courses, therapy, training.

The Tavistock Institue of Human Relations, Belsize Park, London, NW3. Training.

GLOSSARY

Asymmetry   Where one side of the body moves in a different manner from the other.

Body boundary That physical entity from which all perception is recorded and expressed.

Body image The psycho-emotional sense we have of our bodies, related to self-image, formed both by others' feedback to us about our bodies and by our own perception of our bodies.

Body shape The body has a natural capacity to stretch, twist and bend, resulting in shapes which can be, for example, flat, pointed, crooked or rounded.

Centring There is a feeling of balance and inner strength when we are centred. To feel centred is to experience one's psychological centre of gravity, felt in the solar plexus. (See **Hendricks and Wills**, 1975.)

Diagonals These are combinations of left/right and backward/forward (eg. right forward) with levels high and low. For example, left forward high to right backward low, or vice versa; both possible with each side of the body leading the movement.

Dimensions of space When we move in a direction (left/right/forward/backward) and also in a high or low level, dimensions are the result. These lead to movements of closing and opening, advancing and retreating, rising and sinking.

Grounding A basic trust of one's body and a sound relationship to gravity. Misuse of or interference with our essential natures leads to frustration and dissatisfied separation from our bodily ground. (See **Keleman**, 1981.)

Levels Three levels, high, medium and low. High is the furthest point one can reach from the joint from which the movement is activated in gesture (eg. with arms or legs). Medium level is when, eg. the leg is used at hip level, high when it is above the hips, and low when below the hips. With the arm the reference point is the shoulder. The action of stepping would be high if on the toes, medium if on whole sole of foot, and low if done with bent knees.

Locomotion (*See Travelling*)

Pathways We can move in straight, angular or twisted ways in our own personal space, creating different patterns, whether with whole body or gestures of arms, legs etc. These pathways are in the air around us, in general space. Moving over the floor we also create patterns in straight, angular or twisted pathways which create a floor pattern.

Perseveration Repetitive movement which leads nowhere, eg. turning a tap on and off. Often found in disturbed clients.

Populations   This refers to the client groups which may be found in need of special care and intervention, for example, the learning disabled or psychiatric populations.

Rebirthing   Rebirthing itself is seen as a spiritual discipline where the birth experience is re-lived. Sometimes the process of initiating the birthing movement patterns triggers deeply repressed birth memories, and re-activates the primal struggle to live or die. Primal therapy in particular can assist in integrating these experiences.

Relationship   This implies initiating, maintaining, rejecting, ignoring contact. It involves listening, watching or responding to contact, whether visual, verbal, tactile, kinaesthetic or auditory, with others, objects, or the space.

Ritual   An often repeated series of actions; a performance of rites; a body or code of ceremonies. This could be, for example, the group's agreed and intentional convention, such as how the session starts and finishes.

Symmetry   Movement where both sides of the body move in the same manner/shape at the same time.

Travelling/locomotion   Form of stepping in general space. Going from one place to another in a transference of weight.

Underbounded   Where the individual is lacking in containment; much free flow of movement as in hyperactivity or flaccidity.

JOURNALS

Changes — Journal of Psychology and Psychotherapy, Jenny Firth Cozens, Department of Clinical Psychology, University of Leicester, Leicester LE1 7RH.

Dance Theatre Journal, Laban Centre for Movement and Dance, Laurie Grove, New Cross, London SE24.

Human Potential Magazine, 5 Layton Road, London N1 0PX.

Journal of Arts in Psychotherapy, 20 Ridgecrest East, Scarsdale, NY 10583, USA (commissioning editor for Dance Movement Therapy, UK, is Bonnie Meekums, 121 Wide Lane, Morley, Leeds, LS27 8DB).

Journal of the ADTA, Suite 230, 2000 Century Plaza, Columbia, Maryland 21044 USA.

New Dance Magazine, 64–84, Chisenhale Road, London E3 5PZ.

Self and Society — Journal of the Association for Humanistic Psychology, 39 Blenkarne Road, London SW11 6HZ.

It is useful to develop for yourself a wide repertoire of resources. The following are some suggestions.

Equipment

Little is needed to practise in a 'barefoot' sense, apart from a suitable space. However, the following are useful:

(a) tape player;
(b) a selection of music tapes;
(c) props such as elastic, parachute, material, mats;
(d) percussion;
(e) sheets of drawing paper and felt-tips or crayons.

Source books

These books are useful for delving into for further information and materials, and are less academic in nature than the sources cited in the bibliography.

Baldwin F and Whitehead M, *That Way and This*, Chatto & Windus, London, 1972.

Benson JF, *Working more Creatively with Groups*, Tavistock, London, 1987.

Bond T, *Games for Social and Life Skills*, Hutchinson, London, 1986.

Bradling R, *Festive Occasions in the Primary School*, Ward Lock, London, 1981.

Brandes D, *Gamesters Handbook II*, Hutchinson, London, 1984.

Cheney G and Strader J, *Modern Dance*, Allyn and Bacon, Boston, 1975.

Ernst S and Goodison L, *In Our Own Hands: a Book of Self-Help Therapy*, The Women's Press, London, 1981.

Groves L (Ed), *Physical Education for Special Needs*, Cambridge University Press, 1979.

Holle B, *Motor Development in Children: Normal and Retarded*, Blackwell Scientific Publications, Oxford, 1981.

Huang A, *Embrace Tiger, Return to Mountain: the Essence of T'ai Chi*, Real People Press, Moab, Utah, 1973.

Levete G, *No Handicap to Dance*, Souvenir Press, London, 1982.

Parratt AL, *Indoor Games and Activities*, Hodder & Stoughton, London, 1983.

Pierce-Jones F, *The Alexander Technique: Body Awareness in Action*, Schosken Books, New York, 1976.

Shreeves R, *Children Dancing,* Ward Lock Educational, London, 1979.

Stokes EM, *Word Pictures as a Stimulus for Creative Dance,* MacDonald & Evans, London, 1970.

Totton N and Edmondson E, *Reichian Growth Work,* Prism Press, Dorset, 1988.

Upton G (Ed), *Physical and Creative Activities for the Mentally Handicapped,* Cambridge University Press, 1979.

White T, *Visual Poetry for Creative Interpretation,* MacDonald & Evans, London, 1969.

Wosien M, *Sacred Dance: Encounter with the Gods,* Thames and Hudson, London, 1974.

Other areas to explore in books could be stories, mythology and science fiction. For background reading to the Arts and Disabilities:

The Attenborough Report (1985), Carnegie UK Trust, Bedford Square Press.

After Attenborough (1988), Carnegie UK Trust, Bedford Square Press.

There is a database for Europe on Arts and Disabilities at Hertfordshire College of Art and Design.

The use of music

First a word about the limitations in using music. One of the greatest problems when using pre-recorded music with your groups is that the movement may need to change in its quality or rhythm but the music will continue to impose its essential phrasing etc. This could impede the group's creativity and distract from the group development and process. Music cannot respond to the immediacy of individual and group emotion, although it may be selected purposely to pre-empt, contradict or reflect emotional states present in the group. Some groups may become dependent upon the music, being unable to motivate themselves, with the resulting loss in spontaneity. Familiar music may stimulate past memories and perhaps have specific phenomena associated with it which could negatively or positively influence the group. Music can be too controlling, especially if the leader is the only person in the group to select it. It can also dictate the mood, the rhythm, the movement and the energy level for the group. This may result in a repression or an ignoring of fundamental needs. Although these factors may be entirely appropriate for your particular group and the aims/objectives you have set, you will need to be familiar with the music in your resource bases and to be clear why you are using it. An understanding of music's powerful qualities and its advantages and disadvantages at different stages of your group's life can free you and your group.

The choice of music is very personal. Whatever motivates you to dance is usually a useful guideline. Music may be used in many ways, for example:

1   The dance may follow the construction of the music which has a *shaping* emphasis and a repetition of the same theme, eg. *Monotones* by Erik Satie, or as in a fugue. It may suggest different people moving at different times or different groups of people. One person may follow the theme, whilst others accompany with smaller/bigger variations on their dance movements.

2   The dance could be based on the mood or feeling — the tone of the music, that is, it could be interpreted emotionally, eg. Bessie Smith 'Blues' songs, *Star Wars* theme tune.

3   The dance could be a reaction to the action and rhythm of the music eg. Mussorsky *Pictures at an Exhibition*, Gnome section.

4   The music could set an atmosphere for a dance drama, eg. *Echoes* by Emerson, Lake and Palmer or *War of the Worlds*. The movement will still need to follow the climax, change, increases and decreases, pauses in the music, however.

5   Individual instruments may be followed in the dance, giving variety and relationship to a group dance.

When using music for interpretation it is important that the piece be short, especially for those with limited attention spans. Select a piece that you know well enough to fade out at a given place. It could be pre-recorded with a fade. You may need to allow time in the session to rehearse dances without accompaniment.

Music can be used as a *stimulus motivator* or as an *accompaniment* for the dance. If working with live musicians, a piece of music can be composed as the dance is made, or following the choreography of the piece. Percussion may be used after the dance has been created in a similar manner. Pre-recorded music can also be added afterwards, although the shape of the dance will have to be adapted in places.

Music may be used at any point during the session to accompany warm-up activities, creative work or a completed dance. One piece or two contrasting pieces may be used. It may be good for safety, encouraging movement and relaxing inhibitions, for some groups. Below are a few selections from music (pre-recorded) which have been found to be useful. The list is not intended to be comprehensive.

General

Andrews Sisters — any appropriate
Blue Danube — Strauss
Blue — Otis Reading
Brandenburg Concertos — London Philharmonic Orchestra
Capriccio Espagnol and Scheherazade — Rimsky-Korsakov
Carnival of the Animals — Saint-Saëns
Children Dancing (tape) — R. North-Ward Lock Educational
Dancing Circles, Tape I — Colin Harrison, PO Box 26, Glastonbury, Somerset, BA6 9YA
Ghost Dances — The Mercury Ensemble (South American) Folk Songs. Arranged Nicholas Carr courtesy of Inti-illimani
Graceland — Paul Simon
Greatest Hits — Paul Simon
Guitar Recital — John Williams and *Cavatina/Romanza* by John Williams
La Flute Indienne — Los Calchakis et Los Gaucharacos
Lord of the Rings — Bo Hanson
Magic Windows — Herbie Hancock
Midnight Express — Film soundtrack
New World Cassettes, PO Box 15, Twickenham TW1 4SP (eg. *Crystal Dancer* by Phil Wells).
Music for Dance Class (tape) — Available from C. Benstead, 42 Lincoln Road, London N29 DL at £6.75
On Broadway — George Benson
Piano Rags (The Entertainer) — Scott Joplin
Pictures at an Exhibition — Mussorgsky
Playground on Mars (*Chariots of Fire*) — Title track
Polestar — Vangelis
Ritual Fire Dance — De Falla
Ry Cooder — any
Snowflakes are Dancing — Tomita
Switched on Bach
Toyshop from *The Sorcerer's Apprentice*, Paul Dukas
Variations — Andrew Lloyd Webber
Water Music — Handel

Stepping (warming-up)

Architecture and Morality — Orchestral Manoeuvres in the Dark
Borodin, Palovtsian Dances from Prince Igor — Rimsky-Korsakov and Glazunov

Cacharpaya — Incantations
Dave Brubeck's Greatest Hits — CBS
Dawn — Steve Halpern (Halpern Sounds, 1775 Old Country Rd #9, Belmont, CA 94002, USA)
Dr Who Theme — BBC Records
Favourite Piano Pieces — Chopin, Decca
The Flight of the Condor — BBC Records
Fragile — Yes
Golliwogs' Cakewalk — Mussorgsky
Hall of the Mountain King — Grieg
Jungle Rhythms and Chants — Olympic Records
The Light of Experience — Gheorghe Zamfir
Music from India No. 10 — Imrat Kahn
One Step Beyond — Madness
Oxygen — Jean-Michael Jarre
Pizzicato Polka, Circus, Tritsch-Tratsch Polka — Strauss
The Planets Suite — Holst
2001, a Space Odyssey — MGM Records

Light and fun (warm-up)

Bach — any appropriate
Chopin — Any piano pieces
Floral Dance — Brighouse and Rastrick Brass Band
Match of the Day (theme tune) — Tony Osborne
Mikrokosmos — Bartok
Vivaldi — any appropriate

Dreamy blues

Ain't Misbehavin' — Fats Waller (RCA)
Drinking Rum and Coca-Cola — Andrews Sisters
God Bless the Child — Billie Holiday
Healing Tapes from New Age Music
Midnight Cowboy — Bob Dylan
Singing the Blues — J.J. Cale

Step patterns and rhythms

Music of Mikis Theodorikis (Zorba's Dance)
Thriller (The Beat) — Michael Jackson
Tijuana Brass Albums

Stately, regular

Gymnopedies 1, 2 & 3 — Erik Satie (from Monotones)

Historical Dance Music
Largo — Handel
Pomp and Circumstance, Clockwork Orange film theme

Quick and exciting

Baggy Trousers — Madness
National Folk Dance Records
Zip-a-dee-do-Dah — Mickey Mouse Disco

Dramatic (could follow story line)

Bang on a Drum — BBC Records, cassette MRMC 004 and cassettes
BBC Radiophonic Music (Series) REC 25
March of Dwarfs — Grieg, Lyric Suite, Op. 54
Moving Percussion and Electronic Sound Pictures L & M D4
Piano Man — Billy Joel
Sound Effects, BBC Records No. 3, RED 102 M
'Voices' Four records, First Book (poems, songs, music) Argo DA 91

Shaping dances

Begegnungen — Eno, Moebius, Roedelius, Plank
Bolero — Ravel
Fingal's Cave — Mendelssohn
The Good, the Bad and the Ugly (theme) — Morricone
Le Cygne — Saint Saëns
Masters of Irish Music — Martin Byrnes
New World Symphony — Dvorak
Peer Gynt, Morning — Grieg
Prelude à L'Après-Midi d'un Faune — Debussy
World of Mozart — Mozart

Strength and atmosphere

Cantavina — John Williams
Sky — I and II (Ariola Records)
Slip Slidin' Away — Paul Simon

Soft feeling tones

Albatross — Fleetwood Mac
Circles — New Seekers
Nocturne Op. 15 no. 2 — Chopin
Waltz No. 14 — Chopin

You will need to listen to a wide range of music. Remember it is the synthesis of the movement and the music which is exciting, showing the shape of the phrase and the flow of the music. The best way to form ideas and impressions of the use of music is to see other people's approaches to the problem. It is desirable to get to live performances of music and dance as much as possible. All major dance companies have education officers who will inform you of local opportunities for seeing their company perform. There are many companies who see their role as educating in dance as an art form and who will visit your setting for workshops and performances.

REFERENCES

Allport GW, *Pattern and Growth in Personality,* Holt, Rinehart & Winston, New York, 1961.

Bainbridge G, Duddington A, Collingdon M and Gardner C, 'Dance-Mime: A contribution to treatment in Psychiatry', *Journal of Mental Science,* 99, pp 308–14, 1953.

Birdwhistell R, *Kinesics and Context,* University of Pennsylvania Press, Philadelphia, 1970.

Blacking J, *Anthropology of the Body,* Academic Press, London, 1977.

Chace M, *Marion Chace; Her Papers* (ed Chaiklin H) American Dance Therapy Association, 1975.

Cohen SJ (Ed), *The Modern Dance,* Wesleyan University Press, Middletown, Connecticut, 1966.

Condon W, *Linguistic Kinesic Research and Dance Therapy,* Proceedings, 3rd Annual Conference, ADTA, 1969.

Curl G, 'A Critical Study of Rudolf von Laban's Theory and Practice of Movement', MEd thesis, University of Leicester, 1967.

Doyne *et al.*, 'Running versus Weightlifting in the Treatment of Depression', *Journal of Consulting and Clinical Psychology* 55, pp 748–54, 1987.

Espenak L, *Dance Therapy — Theory and Application,* Charles Thomas, Springfield, Illinois, 1981.

Foster J, *The Influences of Rudolf Laban,* Lepus Books, London, 1977.

Gendlin E, *Experiencing and the Creation of Meaning,* New York Free Press, Glencoe, 1962.

Gulbenkian Foundation, *Dance Education and Training in Britain* (ed Brinson P) London, 1980.

Hall ET, *The Silent Language,* Doubleday Press, New York, 1973.

Heinicke C and Westheimer I, *Brief Separations,* Longman, London, 1966.

Hendricks G and Wills K, *The Centering Book*, Spectrum Books, Prentice-Hall, New Jersey, 1975.

Keleman S, *Your Body Speaks its Mind*, Center Press, California, 1981.

Laban R, *Modern Educational Dance*, Macdonald & Evans, Plymouth, 1978.

Laban R, 'Some Notes on Movement Therapy', *Laban Guild Magazine* 71, pp 19–20, 1983.

Lamb W and Watson E, *Body Code: The Meaning in Movement*, Routledge & Kegan Paul, London, 1979.

Leste A and Rust J, 'Effects of Dance on Anxiety', *Journal of Perceptual and Motor Skills* 58, pp 767–72, 1984.

Levete G, *No Handicap to Dance*, Souvenir Press, London, 1985.

May P, Wexler M, Falkin J and Schoop T, 'Non-verbal Techniques in the Reestablishment of Body Image and Self-id-entity — A Report', in **Costonis MN (Ed)**, *Therapy in Motion*, University of Illinois Press, Chicago, 1978.

Meekums B, 'Family Dance Therapy', *New Dance* 41, pp 6–8, 1987.

North M, *Personality Assessment Through Movement*, Macdonald & Evans, Plymouth, 1972.

Oliver N, 'Recreation for the severely mentally handicapped', *Proceedings Third Symposium of the Joseph P. Kennedy Jnr. Foundation, Boston, Expanding Concepts in Mental Retardation*, 1968.

Oliver N, 'Physical Activity and the Psychological development of the Handicapped', in **Kane JE (Ed)**, *Psychological Aspects of Physical Education and Sport*, Routledge & Kegan Paul, London, 1975.

Payne HL, 'Movement Therapy in a Special Educational Setting', *Cambridge Institute of Education, Conference Proceedings — Current Developments in Special Education*, 1979.

Payne (West) HL, 'The Development of the Association for Dance Movement Therapy', *New Dance* 27, Autumn/Winter, pp 17–19, 1983.

Payne (West) HL, 'Responding with Dance', *Maladjustment and Therapeutic Education* 2, 2, pp 42–57, 1984.

Payne HL, 'Perceptions of Male Adolescents Labelled Delinquent towards a Programme of Dance Movement Therapy', unpublished MPhil thesis, University of Manchester, 1987.

Payne HL, 'The Use of Dance Movement Therapy with Troubled Youth', in **Schaefer CE (Ed)**, *Innovative Interventions in Child and Adolescent Therapy*, John Wiley, New York, 1988.

Piaget J, *Origins of Intelligence in Childhood*, Routledge & Kegan Paul, 1952.

Pirsig RM, *Zen and the Art of Motorcycle Maintenance*, Corgi, London, 1976.

Puretz SL, 'Influence of Modern Dance on Body Image', *Essays in Dance Research, Dance Research Annual,* IX, pp 13–30, CORD, New York, 1978.

Rogers C, *On Becoming a Person,* Constable, London, 1971.

Sachs C, *The World History of Dance,* Norton and Co, New York, 1937.

Sandle JN, 'Aesthetics and the Psychology of Qualitative Movement', in **Kane JE (Ed),** *Psychological Aspects of Physical Education and Sport,* Routledge & Kegan Paul, London, 1975.

Schilder P, *The Image and Appearance of the Human Body,* International Universities Press, New York, 1950.

Schoop T, *Won't You Join the Dance?,* Mayfield Publishers, Palo Alto, 1973.

Sherborne V, 'Building Relationships through Movement with Children with Communication Problems', *Inscape* 1, 10, British Association of Art Therapists, 1974.

Stern D, *The First Relationship — Infant and Mother,* Fontana/Open Books, London, 1979.

Stern D, *The Interpersonal World of the Infant,* Basic Books, New York, 1985.

Wethered A and Gardner C, in **Burr L (Ed),** *Therapy through Movement,* Nottingham Rehabilitation, Nottingham, 1986.

BIBLIOGRAPHY

Bartenieff I and Lewis D, *Body Movement: Coping with the Environment,* Gordon & Breach Science Publishers, London, 1980.

Bartenieff I, 'How is the Dancing Teacher equipped to do Dance Therapy?', *ADTA Monographs No. 1,* Columbia.

Bate R, Weir M and Parker C, *Movement and Growth Programmes for the Elderly and Those Who Care for Them,* ADMT Publications, London, 1985.

Boadella D, *Lifestreams: An Introduction to Biosynthesis,* Routledge & Kegan Paul, London, 1987.

Bowlby J, *The Making and Breaking of Affectional Bonds,* Tavistock, London, 1979.

Caplow-Lindner E et al., *Therapeutic Dance Movement: Expressive Activities for Older Adults,* Human Sciences Press, New York/London, 1979.

Casement P, *On Learning From the Patient,* Tavistock Publications, London & New York, 1985.

Bainbridge-Cohen B and Mills M, *Developmental Movement Therapy, ADMT Publications, London, 1979.*

Costonis MN, *Therapy in Motion,* University of Illinois Press, London, 1978.

Dell C, *A Primer for Movement Description,* Dance Notation Bureau, New York, 1970.

Erikson E, *Childhood and Society,* Penguin, Harmondsworth, 1978.

Feder E and B, *The Expressive Arts Therapies: Art, Music and Dance as Psychotherapy,* Prentice-Hall, New Jersey, 1981.

Ferrucci P, *What We May Be. An Introduction to Psychosynthesis,* Northamptonshire Turnstone Press, 1982.

Fisher S and SE Cleveland, *Body Image and Personality,* Dover, New York, 1968.

Gellhorn E, 'Motion and Emotion: The Role of Proprioception in the Philosophy and Pathology of the Emotions', *Psychological Review,* 71 pp 457–72, 1964.

Gendlin E, 'Focusing', *Journal of Psychotherapy, Research and Practice 6, pp 4–15, 1962.*

Hanna JL, *To Dance is Human. A Theory of Non-verbal Communication,* University of Texas Press, Austin/London, 1979.

Harris JG, *A Practicum for Dance Therapy,* ADMT Publications, London, 1984.

Jennings S (Ed), *Creative Therapy,* Pitman, London, 1973.

Jung CG, *Man and His Symbols,* Penguin, Harmondsworth, 1964.

Kestenberg J, 'The Role of Movement, Patterns in Development', *Psychoanalytic Quarterly,* XXXVI, 1967.

Laban R, *The Mastery of Movement,* Macdonald & Evans, Plymouth, 1975.

Lefco H, *Dance Therapy: Narrative Case Histories of Therapy Sessions with Six Patients,* Nelson Hall, Chicago, 1973.

Leventhal Marcia, *Movement & Growth: Dance Therapy for the Special Child,* New York University Press, New York, 1980.

Levy F, *Dance/Movement Therapy: A healing art,* NDA/AAHPERD, Virginia, 1988.

Lewis P (Ed), *Theory and Methods in Dance Movement Therapy,* Kendall/Hunt Publishing, Iowa, 1972.

Lewis P (Ed), *Theoretical Approaches in Dance Movement Therapy,* vol 1, Kendall/Hunt Publishing, Iowa, 1979.

Lewis P (Ed), *Theoretical Approaches in Dance Movement Therapy,* vol 2, Kendall/Hunt Publishing, Iowa, 1984.

Lowen A, *The Language of the Body,* Collier Macmillan, London, 1971.

Mason KC (Ed), *Focus on Dance VII — Dance Therapy,* American

Association of Health, Education & Recreation, Washington DC, 1974.

McNiff S, *The Arts and Psychotherapy,* Charles Thomas, Springfield, Illinois, 1981.

Moore C, *Executives In Action,* Macdonald & Evans, Plymouth, 1982. (1st edn 1978, entitled *Action Profiling*).

Payne HL, 'Jumping for Joy', *Changes — Journal for Psychology and Psychotherapy,* vol 3, no.3, 1985.

Payne HL (Ed), *Dance Movement Therapy: Theory and Practice,* Tavistock/Routledge, London, 1992.

Preston-Dunlop V, *A Handbook for Modern Educational Dance,* Macdonald Evans, London, 1963.

Sacks O, *The Man who Mistook His Wife for a Hat,* Picador, Pan Books, London, 1985.

Saltzberger-Wittenberg I, *Psychoanalytic Insight and Relationships,* Routledge & Kegan Paul, London, 1970.

Scheflen AE, with Scheflen A, *Body Language and The Social Order,* Prentice-Hall, Englewood Cliffs, New Jersey, 1972.

Schilder P, *The Image and Appearance of the Human Body,* International Universities Press, New York, 1955.

Schoop T, with Mitchell P, *Won't You Join the Dance: A Dancer's Essay into the Treatment of Psychosis,* National Press Books, Palo Alto, California, 1974.

Schwartz-Salant N and Stein M (Eds), *The Body in Analysis,* Chiron, Illinois, 1986.

Siegal E, *Dance Movement Therapy. Mirror of Our Selves: The Psychoanalytic Approach,* Human Sciences Press, New York/ London, 1984.

Silbermann L (Ed), *Dance Therapy Bibliography,* American Dance Therapy Association, Columbia, 1984.

Spencer P, *Society and the Dance,* Cambridge University Press, 1986.

Todd ME, *The Thinking Body,* Dance Horizons Inc, New York, 1932 (7th printing 1979).

Warren B (Ed), *Using Creative Arts in Therapy,* Croom Helm, London, 1984.

Wethered A, *Drama and Movement in Therapy,* Macdonald & Evans, London 1973.

Winnicott DW, *Playing and Reality,* Penguin Tavistock Publications, London, 1974.

Youngerman S, 'Curt Sachs and His Heritage. A Critical Review of World History of the Dance', *Dance Research Journal 6:2,* pp 6–19, 1974.

Zukav G, *The Dancing Wu Li Masters,* Fontana, London, 1979.

INDEX TO ACTIVITIES